Early Childhood Deafness

edited by

Ellen Kurtzer-White and David Luterman

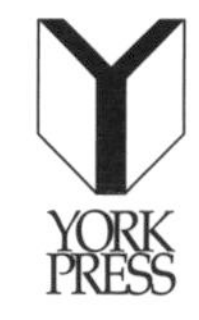

York Press, Inc.
Baltimore

This book was manufactured in the United states of America.

Typography by Type Shoppe II Productions, Ltd.
Printing and binding by Data Reproductions Corp.
Cover design by Joseph Dieter, Jr.

Library of Congress Cataloging-in-Publication Data

Early childhood deafness / edited by Ellen Kurtzer-White and David Luterman.
p. cm.
Includes bibliographical references and index.
ISBN 0-912752-61-0 (pbk.)
1. Deafness in children--Congresses. 2. Hearing disorders in children--Congresses. I. Kurtzer-White, Ellen. II. Luterman, David.
RF291.5.C45 E27 2001
618.92'0978--dc21 2001040145

Early Childhood Deafness

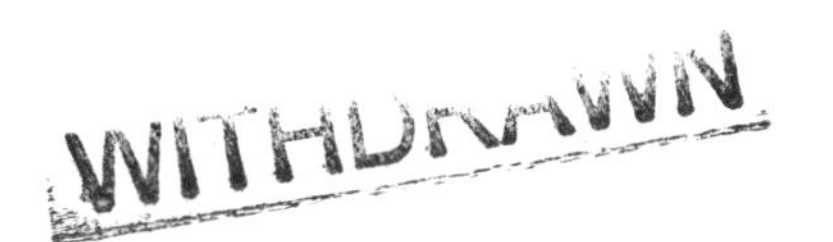

Contents

Preface

For the five years I supervised the Thayer Lindsley Nursery at Emerson College, two questions were raised at the beginning of each academic year. Inevitably, the first was "Can you believe those Red Sox?" (particularly when they were losing) quickly followed by "When is Luterman finally going to retire?" There was some congruity to those questions. Both were posed rhetorically, with good humor, and the expectation that we would all ask them again the next year. But David finally gave the faculty a response as incredulous as the Red Sox winning the World Series; he would retire in 2000. Although we all knew intellectually that this day would come, colleagues at Emerson, families in our programs, students and professionals alike could not and probably did not want to imagine what life would be like without David lumbering down the halls of 216 Tremont Street. I think David would have called this the shock and denial phase of our grief response. We all felt a loss.

David has been a remarkable force and influence in work with families of children with hearing loss and has touched professionals and parents with his scholarship, publications, classes and workshops. In deference to my mentor, I am not going to review his impressive list of credentials and achievements. Rather, I am going to transcend that "informational content" to go to the emotional reality that is at the heart of David's career. David Luterman is loved and respected, and as Fred Bess once said to me, "He (David) really defines the word mensch." Families return to Emerson 30 years after their initial contact, when they first began their journey into deafness, their toddlers now adults with careers and families of their own. Former students write from around the country that they are trying to recreate the supportive and nurturing environment they experienced here within their own workplaces. For me personally, he has been a mentor and dear friend.

For those of us who have worked with him, David is somewhat of an enigma: a tenured professor who is just now beginning to use a computer—all previous manuscripts have been scratched in long hand at his kitchen table; the founder and director of Thayer Lindsley Nursery, who by his own admission is terrified of being left alone in a room with a two-year old, yet is undaunted by what most professionals find much more terrifying—working with families who are struggling to face the emotional challenges resulting from the diagnosis of early childhood hearing loss; a soft spoken man whose words are powerful enough to be heard in Japan, New Zealand, Zimbabwe, Australia, and Scotland.

David is many things to us; friend, colleague and counselor. He is the voice that reminds us that stressful situations and life events are catalysts for growth and change, to pay attention to parents emotional well-being and mental health as well as our own. David has a trademark saying, "Deafness is a great teacher." How fortunate we have been to have him teach us that message. It is with these lessons in mind that this symposium was convened, to honor a truly great teacher and to celebrate David's new status of professor emeritus.

Ellen Kurtzer-White

Introduction

Within a compressed time period, there have been remarkable, revolutionary changes in the field of audiology that have had a significant impact on families and their young children with hearing loss and that demand professionals to rethink diagnostic and intervention paradigms. The Thayer Lindsley Family Centered Nursery at Emerson College has felt the impact of these changes as have programs for infants and toddlers with hearing loss throughout the country, if not the world. With Massachusetts joining the growing list of states with legislated universal hearing screening, there has been a need to increase services for infants. Two-year olds are now the senior citizens of our program. With advances in cochlear implant technology and changing candidacy criteria, 100% of the deaf toddlers enrolled in Thayer Lindsley were implanted by the end of the summer of 2000. For those children who benefit from more traditional amplification, we see the youngest nursery members using advanced programmable and digital technology. Families now have more program options to explore. Many have enrolled in American Sign Language (ASL) family learning programs and have become keenly aware of the issues of Deaf pride and culture, while also investigating oral education. As a clinical training program for graduate students in speech language pathology, we have had to rethink what it means to "do therapy" with such very young children and their families. As a result, our curriculum has been revised to better develop students' knowledge base and clinical skills with infant and prelinguistic development. Yet, with all these technological advances and reconceptualized intervention approaches, one thing has remained constant. As professionals, we need to develop our own capacities to meet the needs of parents and families as they make their way through a difficult, emotional and, we hope, joyful journey of parenting a child with hearing loss.

The need to share current research and perspectives on the extraordinary changes and trends in pediatric audiology, early intervention and the education of the deaf was evident. Additionally, we could not think of a more appropriate way to honor David Luterman's contributions to the field and to celebrate his new professor emeritus status than by convening an outstanding faculty for a two-day symposium. The sequence of the presentations (and the chapters of this book) was carefully designed to follow the process from newborn hearing screening to intervention. Mark Ross's seminal work in pediatric audiology, as well as his longstanding relationship as David Luterman's colleague and friend, made him the only choice for the opening remarks. His discussion of history as precursor to the present is timely and thought provoking. Christine Yoshinaga-Itano's name has become synonymous with the topic of universal newborn hearing screening. Her benchmark publications have transformed our anecdotally based beliefs that "earlier is better" to knowledge based on careful and longitudinal research. Dr. Yoshinaga-Itano presents compelling data on the psychosocial implications of newborn hearing screening and diagnosis for parents and the subsequent impact on the child's language development. Universal newborn hearing screening has prompted the need to reconsider diagnostic techniques. Dr. Marilyn Neault, a friend to Thayer Lindsley Nursery and a true advocate for families and children in New England, discusses advances in the diagnostic process and our need to keep that process humane. Dr. Jackson Roush presents data on parental expectations and the need for hope and defined family-centered practice. The potential to fulfill some of the hopes held by parents has geometrically improved over the past several years with advances in technology. Digital and programmable hearing aids, cochlear implants, and wireless FM systems hold the promise of access to a quality speech signal and greater potential for the development of oral language, even for the profoundly deaf infant. Richard Seewald describes systematic, acoustically sound hearing aid fitting strategies for infants, Jane Madell discusses the benefits for assistive listening devices, and Patricia Chute reviews historical developments, and changing candidacy criteria and new developments in cochlear implants.

The technological advances place new demands on the professionals working in this field. The question must be asked, "Has the technology out-paced our ability to plan and implement appropriate intervention?" Attempts to keep current with ever changing, ever improving technical advances can be overwhelming to professionals (and parents). Applying this new technology to very young children and creating sensitive programming for families who are not at all prepared for the diagnosis can be daunting and challenging. Yet, the ultimate outcomes of early identification and the innovative technologies rests with our ability to plan and deliver appropriate intervention that is accessible for all families. Now, more than ever, we must hone our counseling skills and be mindful of incorporating the principle of family centeredness into our professional responsibilities and activities, if we are to contribute positively to the outcomes. Mary Pat Moeller describes the role of the home visitor and the requisite listening/counseling skills that validate parental observation and participation in intervention.

While there has been discussion about the needs of babies and families involved in this process, we must be mindful of the need to create a resource of well trained, empathetic and skillful professionals.

Dr. Fred Bess outlines the changing and expanding list of competencies required of clinicians working with children with hearing loss, and the need for academic institutions to adapt their curricula while encouraging quality research. David Luterman concluded the symposium, and this volume, offering his perspectives on the changes we face.

This collection of papers represents the best contemporary thought on early childhood hearing loss and provides direction for professional development of caring and best-practice intervention.

Ellen Kurtzer-White
David Luterman

CONTRIBUTORS

Fred H. Bess, Ph.D.
Vanderbilt Bill Wilkerson Center for Otolaryngology and Communication Sciences
Vanderbilt University Medical Center
Department of Hearing and Speech Sciences
Nashville, Tennessee
fred.h.bess@vanderbilt.edu

Patricia Chute, Ed.D.
Associate Professor
Mercy College
Department of Communication Disorders
555 Broadway
Dobbs Ferry, New York 10522
pchute@mercynet.edu

Ellen Kurtzer-White, M.S.
Director:
First Connections Resource and Training Project for Newborn Hearing Screening
Rhode Island Department of Health and Rhode Island Department of Education
1 Corliss Park, Providence, RI 02908
ekw@rideaf.net

David Luterman, D.Ed.
Director, The Thayer Lindsley Nursery
Professor Emeritus
Emerson College
120 Boylston Street
Boston, Massachusetts 02116

Mary Pat Moeller, M.S.
Director, Center for Childhood Deafness
Boy's Town National Research Hospital
555 North 30th Street
Omaha, Nebraska 68131
moeller@boystown.org

Jane Madell, Ph,D.
Hearing, Speech and Language Center
Beth Israel Medical Center
Suite 2K
10 Union Square, East
New York, New York 10003

Marilyn Neault, Ph.D.
Director, Audiology
Children's Hospital Medical Center
Longwood Avenue
Boston, Massachusettes
neault@altch.harvard.edu

Mark Ross, Ph.D.
Professor Emeritus
University of Connecticut
9 Thomas Drive
Storrs, Connecticut 06268

Jackson Roush, Ph.D.
Director, Speech and Hearing Services
Division of Speech and Hearing Sciences
University of North Carolina School of Medicine
CO 7190
Chapel Hill, North Carolina 27599
jack.roush@css.unc.edu

Richard Seewald, Ph.D.
Professor
National Center for Audiology
University of Western Ontario
London, Ontario
Canada
seewald@nca.uwo.ca

Christine Yoshinaga-Itano, Ph.D.
University of Colorado-Boulder
Department of Speech, Language and Hearing Sciences
Campus Box 409
Boulder, Colorado 80309-0409
Christie.yoshi@colorado.edu

Chapter ▪ 1

Some Reflection on Early Childhood Deafness

Mark Ross

Looking at the titles of the papers presented in this volume, one might think that little has changed in the past forty years since David Luterman—in whose honor this book is dedicated—first entered the field. We seem to be covering the same ground over and over, if similar titles and themes are any evidence. Well, we are and we aren't. Of course, early detection and management considerations still take center stage, as they should. What's different now, in spite of the similarity in paper titles, is the confluence of new legislative mandates and technological advances that affect both detection and management directly. In other words, we not only know a lot more, but we are also required to do a lot more. In the following pages, we will be reading about what we are now able to do, particularly in regard to newborn screening programs, outcome measures, amplification options, and the impact of the relatively new player in this game, cochlear implants. As we consider these new developments, we should keep in mind that in perhaps the most significant areas of all, very little has changed. What I would like to do in the following pages is reflect both on what I believe has changed in the past forty years and what has not.

PARENTS

What has not changed is the reaction of parents when they are first informed that their child is deaf. Parents still go through the stages of disbelief, denial, anger, and grief that they have always gone through.

For them, this is a one-time, unexpected event, the first time in history it has ever happened—because it's happening to them. Few such parents have had any experience with deaf people. They know nothing about all the age-old controversies, all the choices that they will be asked to make. At this stage, what they have going through their minds is the death of their initial dreams, their groping attempts to come to terms with what they perceive is a tragic reality, and their feelings of complete inadequacy in meeting all the confusing and yet undefined challenges they will have to face. What we must do is help them understand that their child should still be a source of joy and satisfaction, whose future can still be as rich and fulfilling as any hearing child's. This hasn't changed.

What also has not changed is the need for parents to share their feelings with other parents of children with hearing loss. We know that the emotional support that parents can provide each other far exceeds what professionals can provide parents at this time. While this need has always been with us, years ago it was the exception more than the rule for it to be recognized as a vital component of any management program for young hearing-impaired children. This is one area that has changed tremendously in the past forty years, thanks in great part to the work done by David Luterman. For all of this period, through his books, lectures, and clinical work, he has taught us to respect and trust the parents of the children we see in our clinics. If this emphasis seems obvious now, it is in large part because he, and a few other pioneers like him, have done their work so well.

PROFESSIONALS

The need for skilled professionals to work with the children and their parents also has not changed. Such professionals still need specialized training and experience, beyond that offered in the typical Audiology, Speech-Language Pathology, or Education of the Deaf programs. While some of the responsibilities and roles of these three groups overlap and some are in dispute, there should be no dispute regarding the need for a competency-based formulation: anyone who takes on any role with young hearing impaired children must demonstrate the appropriate background training. Clearly, however, the issue here is exactly how "appropriate" is defined. For example, as an audiologist, my definition of "appropriate" is going to be different from that of a teacher of the deaf who routinely advocates American Sign Language (ASL) as the first language for children with hearing loss. You would think that, after all this time, we would be able to reach some kind of consensus regarding the training, background, and skills of the professionals who work with hearing impaired children and their families. From what I see, it does not look as if we have reached this point yet.

Clinicians dealing with parents of hearing impaired children still have to be able to relate to them in a sensitive, compassionate, and honest manner. Can clinicians be trained to be both academically competent and humanly sensitive? I suspect the answer that Dave Luterman would give would be "yes," given his own record of success in providing such training over the past forty years. Nevertheless, no matter how knowledgeable, compassionate, and experienced we may be, no matter how many deaf children we may have seen in our careers, we must always fight the tendency to fall into a routine, management mode. No children and no parents are "routine"; all require our respect as unique human beings. And although, of course, we should take pride and gain satisfaction from our work, at the same time we must accept the humbling notion that this is not about us, but about parents and their children with hearing impairment. No matter what our personal biases are—and we all have them to some extent—we are still required to respect the authority of parents in having the final say regarding the management of their child. Our role is to lay out, as objectively as we can, various educational and communication options.

MANAGEMENT ISSUES

Even though the children we see in our clinics are younger than we have ever seen them before, the management issues they present are exactly the same as they were forty years ago. We still have to ask why we are so focused on early detection and early management. What do we hope to accomplish? What are our goals? These are not trivial questions. They embody an implicit assumption that an untreated hearing loss will have a profound impact on a child's development, but that the usual consequences can be ameliorated with an early and effective management program. Essentially, we are denying the point of view that a profound hearing loss is a "normative" condition akin to ethnicity—else why provide such programs? Rather, we are declaring through our clinical efforts that a hearing loss is a condition that society has a responsibility to address. Which leads me to my next point.

In every area where some sort of therapy is conducted, the clinician must define the condition as precisely as possible. In this instance, because we are working with children who have a hearing loss, we have to address the fundamental fact that this condition varies widely in a number of dimensions. It follows, therefore, that we need to know as much as we can about the type and configuration of the hearing loss, because much of our therapeutic efforts are—or should be—grounded on this information. Of course all children are unique, with different personalities, aptitudes, and possibilities. And of course, we must "tailor" our approach to an individual child; all this is understood. Too often, however, we seem to deal with such children as if they were all alike in the one dimension that has brought them to our attention—the extent and nature of their hearing loss. On the contrary, if we know anything at all about hearing loss, we know that it varies widely between children, in its nature, degree, and configuration. Obviously, therefore, one major component of any early management program has to be a focus on maximizing the use of the residual hearing. Indeed, it is my contention that one of the most important capabilities a child brings to the therapy process is the extent of his or her residual hearing.

RESIDUAL HEARING

Let us pause for a moment to consider residual hearing. We all know what a hearing loss is, and we are aware that a total hearing loss is a relatively rare occurrence. Residual hearing refers to the hearing that remains, rather than the hearing that is lost. It is where we hope to package amplified sound to permit children as much access to the auditory channel as we can. It is the range between a person's thresholds and the highest level of sound pressure appropriate to deliver. I like the term because it has positive rather than negative implications, as it implies that the auditory channel is still capable of making some of its biological contribution to the welfare of the human being.

Obviously the absence of residual hearing does not make anyone incapable of living a rich and fulfilling life—and I really do want to stress this point. However, the sense of hearing ordinarily does play a vital role in human development and interactions. When we think of audition, we most think of the sensory basis for auditory-verbal language development—undoubtedly its most important function. Through many years of research and clinical experience, we know that even a little bit of residual hearing can contribute to communicative and linguistic development. What is less often appreciated, however, is that residual hearing can do more than foster performance in these communicative dimensions.

The auditory sense provides a channel to the brain that not only informs us about the world around us, but also enriches our overall perception of the world. By being immersed in a three-dimensional acoustic sphere, we are able, consciously or unconsciously, to adapt to and feel part of our immediate surroundings. We are able to identify potentially dangerous or significant unseen events because we can "tune in" selectively to the sound waves that surround us. Unlike our eyes, our ears are always "open" to receive stimuli and thus we are able to monitor our surroundings continuously through this auditory connection. Just because someone has a hearing loss does not mean that he or she need be deprived of all the non-linguistic contributions that audition can make. As long as a person possesses any residual hearing at all, some potentially significant sensory information from the auditory channel can still be obtained.

Some of us older folks may recall an auditory hierarchy concept first described by Donald Ramsdell after World War II. After many experiences with newly deafened servicemen, he realized that many of their complaints transcended their evident communication problems, but dealt with, instead, their inability to hear background sounds, sounds that they had not previously been aware of consciously. They would often complain that the world seemed "dead." Ramsdell postulated that their reaction reflected the loss of the lowest level on the hierarchy of hearing, the primitive or background level. He believed that these background sounds served to psychologically "couple" people to the world around them. Although people may not be consciously aware of sounds at this level, the sounds are still present and still being processed by the brain. When some sound event, such as a shouting voice or an emergency vehicle siren, emerges from this background, it would be considered the second stage in Ramsdell's auditory hierarchy, the signaling or warning level of hearing.

I like to consider these two lowest levels as appropriate therapy goals relevant for any child with any degree of residual hearing. This is a point worth emphasizing: Providing children with hearing loss with an auditory connection to the world is a realizable and valuable goal for the overwhelming majority of them. Note that this is not an argument for or against any communication mode for children. It is an assertion that no professional or educator should deny young children a reasonable opportunity to use their residual hearing. To do so imposes one's personal values on a very fundamental sensory inheritance of other human beings.

COCHLEAR IMPLANTS

Of all the changes that have taken place in the last forty years that have had an impact on people with hearing loss, the advent of cochlear implants has to rank as the most portentous. For the first time in history, we are able to provide usable auditory sensations to people with profound and total hearing losses. For the first time, we have a truly auditory option for people for whom we previously had only visual options, either oral or manual. That the device has had a major impact on all people who are professionally or personally involved with hearing impaired children needs no elaboration from me. I cannot recall any development getting more coverage on TV, in all print media, and on the internet. It seems as if hardly a week goes by without some story about this device, most dramatically as it concern young children. What I would like to discuss is its impact on families and on the Deaf community.

In the past few years, there has been quite intensive discussion regarding the consequences of implants in much of the public media, including a thoughtful and continuing exchange in a recent issue of the Hearing Health magazine. These discussions reveal a great fear among many people in the Deaf community, as well as those allied with this community, that the spread of implants means the end of the Deaf community and the Deaf culture. Thousands of children have already been implanted, at earlier and earlier ages, and it seems to be a process that is feeding on itself. The more children there are who receive cochlear implants, the more it becomes a routine clinical procedure, and the more popular and acceptable the procedure becomes. The Deaf community fears, and rightly so, that the cochlear implant is, and will be, draining off many of their potential members. They believe that these children will be lost to them and that the future viability of the community is now uncertain.

This is not a development that can be viewed with moderation and equanimity by those whose lives and lifestyles are inextricably woven into their Deaf identity. It is only in relatively recent years that Deaf people have achieved acceptance in our society—albeit not complete acceptance—and are free to engage in whatever personal, social, vocational, and civic activities they choose. To an amazing extent, many Deaf people have surmounted the impact of their deafness and are able to lead rich and fulfilling lives. From an historical perspective, it was not too many years ago that Deaf people were denied the right to vote, to testify in legal cases, to receive an inheritance, or to acquire an education. It is this very proud history, and the currently hard-won status, that appears to be threatened by the advent of the cochlear implant. From this perspective, the persistent objections to the provision of cochlear implants for children by some members of the Deaf community and their supporters is perfectly understandable. What, for many of us, is a miraculous device, to them is a threat of extinction to the community. Without a community, without a critical mass, how can there be a Deaf culture? To be quite honest, I do believe that these fears are well founded, that the cochlear implant can threaten the future viability of the Deaf community. At the least, it will change it in some presently unforeseen ways.

It seems that reaching some kind of balanced view on this issue may be even more difficult than reconciling the classic oral and manual controversies! Those arguments have been played out for several hundred years with few modifications and little resolution. The difference that implants have wrought in this argument is that results with them far exceed those obtained with the classical visual-oral approach. Implants are enabling many more deaf children to become effective auditory-verbal communicators than in the past. This fact undermines much of the previous, and often well-founded, objection to the traditional visual-oral approach.

This is not an area in which we have the luxury of postponing decisions. It is not an issue that we can continue to debate until somehow the "truth" emerges. It is not just a question of the current reality (i.e., lots of kids are now being implanted) but also of the nature of the auditory system. If the procedure is going to be done at all, then it should be as early as possible. We need to provide a developmental approach to therapy rather than a remedial approach. This means providing auditory-verbal experiences early in a child's life, so that we can take advantage of the normal linguistic developmental patterns as well as preclude the effects of possible auditory sensory deprivation. However, there are some qualifications we should keep in mind when children receive cochlear implants.

First, a cochlear implant is not a panacea. It does not replace a normal ear. No parent should enter this process believing that this device will completely "fix" a child's hearing loss. Second, we still do not have any good way of accurately predicting just how well an individual child will do with an implant. Some do amazingly well, while others do not (just about all, however, can realize some degree of usable auditory access). Third, it is unlikely that the full potential of an implant can be realized without concurrent and appropriate therapy. And fourth, as the previous point implies, everyone concerned with the child, i.e., school, parents, and others, must be fully committed to do whatever is necessary to realize this potential. One cannot provide a child with an implant and wait for the "miracle" to occur.

It is the parents who must choose whether or not their child should be "treated" with a cochlear implant. Of course, they should be informed of all the management options, in as objective and comprehensive a manner as possible. However, the reality of the situation is that the majority of parents will probably select the option they are most familiar with, the one that permits their child to enter their world. Functionally, and this should be made clear to parents, the child will operate as a hard of hearing person rather than someone with perfectly normal hearing. What we cannot do, and what we have no right to do, is to ask parents to make decisions for their child based on what will ensure the future of the Deaf community.

Some Deaf people will argue passionately that they are recommending what is best for a child, that it is the child's interest that is at stake here and not the parents. I do not question the sincerity of these beliefs. What I do question is the conclusion that a child's best interest can be attained by linguistically and psychologically separating the child from his or her natural parents. This argument would have much more force if we were still in the era of single channel, relatively crude cochlear implants, when the most that could be expected was environmental awareness and a modest improvement in speech-reading performance. That is no longer the case. At the current level of technology, most children with implants are capable of auditory-alone comprehension, permitting them to function as hard of hearing people in an auditory-verbal world. And as a hard of hearing person, I can testify to the profound differences between being deaf—depending primarily upon a visual mode of communication—and being hard of hearing—able to employ a primarily auditory-verbal communication mode.

It could be, of course, that I am also describing a rather extreme position, an assumption that children who receive cochlear implants will identify automatically with the hearing world and not the Deaf world. The real world presents many more shades of gray than this polar formulation suggests. Many children who have implants are continuing their education in Total Communication (TC) programs. In the course of it, they learn sign language and, eventually, particularly as they get older, may prefer to identify closely with the Deaf community. That is also a choice, one that they have every right to make for themselves.

The practical therapy question is whether a child can receive the full benefit of a cochlear implant if he or she is exposed consistently and primarily to simultaneous communication in a TC program. Actually, this is the same question that we have asked for many years, but dealing with hearing aids rather than implants. All of us involved in this area have opinions, often expressed stridently and with a great deal of emotion, but with precious little experimental evidence. For myself, I would say, "It depends." If a child is to become a competent language user, he or she must receive linguistic input that is complete and correct. Based on the way I have seen TC practiced for the past thirty years, this has not been happening. Children were not receiving complete and correct oral or sign samples during attempts to deliver complete messages of both simultaneously. We cannot build a competent language user in two modes when the input for both is impoverished and incomplete.

Is it possible to provide a sufficient quantity and quality of auditory-verbal input for a child to reach maximum capabilities in the auditory-verbal mode, and then do the same in a sign mode? I would say "yes," but this argues for an alternate rather than a simultaneous approach, one that provides sufficient exposure in each mode separately. I do believe that there are some children out there, either wearing cochlear implants or hearing aids, who are competent language users in both the oral and sign modes. How many there are and how they arrived at this happy state are not questions we can now answer. We all have anecdotal reports, plus lots of personal observations filtered through our own belief system. What does seem apparent is that children with implants do require an auditory-verbal focus for at least some presently undefined portion of each day. The auditory system has to be stimulated in some unambiguous fashion, the auditory experiences have to be associated with experiential events, in order for maximum auditory-verbal development to occur.

COCHLEAR IMPLANTS AND HEARING AIDS

As demonstrated by numerous research studies, the auditory benefits associated with the proper use of cochlear implants seems incontrovertible. As someone who has recommended and fitted hearing aids on people for more than forty years, I do have to admit to a bit of envy at all the attention implants are getting. I would like to see the same focus on hearing aids with children that we now see with implants. In the entire world, there are perhaps 10,000 children using cochlear implants. Undoubtedly, the number of children who use hearing aids to gain auditory access to the world is very much greater, perhaps 100 times greater. If we look at the literature of the past ten years, however, it is apparent that articles concerning children with implants are at least as numerous as those dealing with children wearing personal hearing aids. This is quite an imbalance.

Does this paucity of professional literature concerning children wearing hearing aids mean that we have answered all the questions regarding personal amplification? That we know what to do and how to do it? That we are able to ensure that every child who receives any type of personal amplification is making the best use of his or her residual hearing? It would be the brave and foolish person indeed who would dare make that assertion! So how do we explain the popularity of cochlear implants? Part of their current popularity is well understood: They can do things for some people that hearing aids cannot. In that, they are truly new and, to my mind, almost miraculous devices. They can make the deaf hear! But another reason for their popularity is the attention the devices have received from the media, combining as they do the wonders of modern technology and medicine with the social issues of identity and community (great for "human interest" stories). Compared to implants, hearing aids appear to be primitive and unglamorous devices that have a history of poor acceptance and success.

I would like to see the same attention that goes into the selection, fitting, and follow-up of implants also be applied to the selection, fitting, and follow-up of hearing aids. This is not to deny that children who have implants need comprehensive and careful services, only that those wearing personal amplification deserve the same attention. In my optimistic moods, I keep thinking that we will see a "trickle down" effect, where children wearing hearing aids will begin to receive the same care as those wearing implants. In my more pessimistic moods, which unfortunately I also think more realistic, I believe that we will still face the same battles we always did in regard to ensuring appropriate amplification for children. This is sad, considering how much more we know now about providing amplified sound for young children than we did forty years ago.

TERMINOLOGY

Cochlear implants are not the only thing that is new in recent years. The way we employ terminology to describe people with hearing loss has also been changing. Ironically, at the same time cochlear implants are threatening to siphon off future members of the Deaf community, its ranks may be increasing because of the influences of terminology on the auditory management of potentially hard of hearing children. Let me explain what I mean by this assertion.

In previous years, the labels "deaf" and "hard of hearing" were most often employed as subcategories of the term "hearing impaired," used generically to refer to anybody with any auditory disorder. Some people objected to the term "hearing impaired" because they thought it had several negative connotations. Some Deaf people did not believe that their auditory status should be characterized as "impaired" when for them it was a normative condition. The fact that they were unable or unwilling to hear was considered a component of their identity, that they were primarily part of a visual and not auditory world. Others objected that the term implied that the *person* was "impaired" rather than the *hearing*, though this was far from the intention of those who employed the term (as I have in numerous publications).

Because of these reasons, and regardless of their merits, this generic use of the label "hearing impaired" now appears to be in disfavor. Now we see the term "deaf and hard of hearing" being employed instead. In part, the term is being used as a substitute generic label, to refer to all people with hearing loss and partly, apparently, to reflect an extension of the original mission of agencies that heretofore only dealt with "deaf" people. Thus, a number of organizations, agencies, and educational institutions at the national, state, and local levels have recently re-labeled themselves to include the term "hard of hearing" as well as "deaf." Local, regional, and national educational programs, from the elementary to the college level, ostensibly are now designed to assist both "deaf and hard of hearing students," while teacher training programs presume to prepare future professionals to teach all students falling into both categories. Even the Alexander Graham Bell Association for the Deaf now includes "hard of hearing" in its title.

Well, so what? Does this label make a difference? I believe it does. There are many educational programs from the elementary to the post-secondary levels that purport to serve both deaf and hard of hearing students. However, many of these programs utilize only one educational philosophy for their students with known hearing loss, regardless of severity. Almost always in these classrooms, a Total Communication (TC) program is the one employed. Although theoretically, hard of hearing children (or those potentially so, given appropriate auditory management) should also receive the auditory access they require in a TC program, in reality the auditory-oral mode is often given short shrift. Because the teacher is simultaneously signing while speaking, the oral language component is rarely complete and grammatical. Hearing aids and auditory training systems are not monitored and sometimes not even used. In some schools that claim to care for both deaf and hard of hearing students, American Sign Language (ASL) with "voice-off" is the instructional language. Although perhaps not explicitly forbidden, the value system developed in such schools often discourages the use of audition.

These are the kinds of educational experiences that, I believe, can and do turn audiologically hard of hearing children into functionally deaf adults. This is where the future recruits to the Deaf community will come from. None of this is malicious, none of it is done without the best of intentions. Leaders of the Deaf community know very little about hearing, though they undoubtedly know quite a bit about its absence. They truly believe that hard of hearing children "belong" to the Deaf community, that they will be happier as part of a visual world than struggling as hard of hearing people in the hearing world. (Again, we see the polarity that so bedevils this issue.) On the contrary, in our educational programs we should be emphasizing the full use of whatever residual hearing children possess, leaving the question of their future social and cultural identity for them to decide when they are ready.

In a way the lumping together of deaf and hard of hearing people is understandable, simply because both deaf and hard of hearing people display auditory deficiencies of some degree or another. In actuality, however, in spite of some overlapping needs and the presence of some people who fall into a "gray" area, these groups are fundamentally very different. Professionals and the public alike must understand that "hard of hearing" is not some subcategory of "deaf," but rather a different disability with its own implications and needs. This is not simply an exercise in academic taxonomy with no real-world implications. How we label an entity often influences treatment; individual differences are easily lost if diagnostic labels are too inclusive. We should not be surprised if audiologically hard of hearing children, labeled or treated as deaf, who attend schools for the deaf and socialize primarily with deaf children, often identify and function as members of the Deaf community. If the services of some agency are designed in fact to respond only to the needs of deaf people, then its mission should be restricted to this population. If an agency purports to care for hard of hearing people as well, then this fact should be explicitly reflected in the services that are offered. What is unsupportable is the deceptive claim that both "deaf and hard of hearing" people are being cared for by an agency or institution when in reality only services appropriate for deaf people are being provided—for all the clients, both deaf and hard of hearing.

TO SUMMARIZE

It is well for us to keep in mind why we are involved with the early detection and management of children with hearing loss. If these activities did not make a difference in a child's ultimate adjustment and performance, we would not be doing them. One consensus we can claim to have reached concerns the need to identify the presence of a hearing loss early in life, that the sooner we enroll children and parents in some kind of therapeutic program, the better off they will be eventually. For the first time in history, we now have both the forces of law and technology on our side. We can identify the children through impressive newborn hearing screening tools, and we can bring to bear the kinds of sophisticated technology that were not even dreamt of years ago. What hasn't changed, however, and what must always remain the highest priority in our activities is the need to be respectful of the parents and the children. What I mean by this is that it has to be their needs that take priority; that it is the parents and ultimately the children who will define and decide their own live's courses; and that our role is not to direct them or to impose our values on them, but to serve as their agents while they work out their own future.

Chapter ▪ 2

Early Identification and Social-Emotional Factors of Children with Hearing Loss and Children Screened for Hearing Loss

Christine Yoshinaga-Itano and
Carolina Abdala de Uzcategui

Universal newborn hearing screening presents new challenges for professionals involved in birthing hospitals, for diagnostic audiologists, and for those individuals who provide early intervention services. This new population of families and their newborns has characteristics that differ dramatically from the previous generation of families requiring professional services. The appropriate counseling of these families may determine whether or not the families and their children are able to benefit optimally from the advantages presented by earlier identification and intervention. Counseling strategies that are appropriate for each of the different sub-populations resulting from the newborn hearing screening programs must be developed. Some of these sub-populations are: (1) children referred for additional screening who ultimately are determined to have normal hearing; (2) children with unilateral hearing loss; (3) children with otitis media that is medically manageable, but indicative of a high probability of chronic middle ear problems in early childhood; (4) children with auditory neuropathy; (5) children with borderline hearing loss; (6) children with mild to moderate hearing loss; and (7) any child identified with bilateral sensorineural hearing loss within the first few months of life.

Most of the focus of the benefits of early identification and early intervention have been on the language development of early-identified children. Children who have been identified with hearing loss and who receive immediate intervention services during the first six months of life have significantly better language development in the first three years of life (Yoshinaga-Itano et al. 1998) than children identified after six months of age. A critical question concerns what factors besides the age of identification of the hearing loss and the initiation of intervention, predict optimal language development. The issue of successful outcomes for deaf and hard-of-hearing children should not be simplified to these two variables of simply identification of the hearing loss and initiation of intervention.

Early-identified, screened children have better speech ability than later-identified children. Professionals in hearing tend to focus first on access to auditory stimulation. However, from an auditory stimulation perspective, the outcomes measured thus far are not attributable solely to audition. Although several studies have found significantly better speech ability of early-identified and screened children when compared to later-identified and non-screened children (Yoshinaga-Itano and Apuzzo 1998a; Yoshinaga-Itano and Apuzzo 1998b; Yoshinaga-Itano, Coulter, and Thomson 2001), early identification is a variable that creates an opportunity for better speech ability, but is not the primary predictor of speech ability.

Children with mild through profound hearing loss have similar speech characteristics in the first year of life. Surprisingly, even when children have early-identified hearing loss with immediate access to amplification, their speech production in the first year of life is not differentiated by degree of hearing loss from mild through profound (Wallace, Menn, and Yoshinaga-Itano 2000). Children with mild hearing loss have babble that is more similar to children with profound hearing loss than to children with normal hearing in the first twelve months of life, even when hearing loss is identified early. Children with any degree of hearing loss have babble that is significantly different from children with normal hearing even when the hearing loss is identified early. These findings lead to a hypothesis that there may be a threshold of hearing in utero necessary for the normal development of speech in the first year of life. Perhaps early identification and intervention, even at two months of life, are not sufficient to compensate for hearing loss in utero within the first nine to twelve months of life. Neither the presence of babble similar to children with normal hearing nor the absence of babble predict speech outcome. Children with no babble in the first twelve months can develop intelligible speech within the early childhood period. Children with babble similar to that of children with normal hearing may fail to develop intelligible speech.

Age, expressive language, and degree of hearing loss are the primary predictors of speech outcome in the second through sixth years of life. From the second year (12 months) through sixth years of life (71 months), age, language, and degree of hearing loss are the primary predictors of speech outcome (Yoshinaga-Itano and Sedey 2000). Non-verbal cognitive development and age of identification are the primary predictors of expressive language development (Yoshinaga-Itano et al. 1998). Once the variance accounted for by the variables age, expressive language, and degree of hearing loss was analyzed, no additional variance was found for age of identification, indicating that the role of age of identification in speech outcome is the impact on language development.

Several possible factors may be related to the finding that even when identified early and amplified early, children with hearing loss, regardless of degree of hearing loss, have very different speech development than children with normal hearing throughout early childhood. Earmold replacement typically is required at four to six week intervals within the first year of life. The financial resources of the family and ability of the family to maintain a regular audiological follow-through program have a significant impact upon the regular amplification use of the child. Even with regular audiological follow-through, the problems of feedback with amplification are troublesome. Since the infants spend much of their early life nursing and sleeping, feedback problems are the most frequent complaints of families with newly diagnosed children. The priorities of any family with a newborn baby are bonding, enjoying the infant, caring for the essential needs of the baby, and attempting to regain some regularity in the daily family routine. Auditory stimulation, even if the family already has knowledge and skill concerning what to do, are reportedly not the primary focus of the family. Professionals providing this initial intervention report that they spend the vast proportion of their time counseling the family and providing educational information.

However, research on the development of deaf and hard-of-hearing children indicates that the relationship between early identification/intervention on the social-emotional factors of the parent and child are significant. This chapter will discuss these relationships and include the intervention strategies that have been used in the training of professionals providing parent-infant services.

COUNSELING STRATEGIES

Luterman (1987, 1995) has been a primary voice in the focus on counseling strategies that assist families in resolving their grieving from the diagnosis of the hearing loss. The literature contains information that describes emotions expressed by parents about their grieving process (Luterman, Kurtzer-White, and Seewald 1999).

From an intervention perspective, professionals working with families and their young deaf and hard-of-hearing children have reported that a significant amount of time in intervention is spent on assisting families through a process of grief or mourning after the diagnosis of hearing loss. Children with a hearing loss identified early differ from children identified later because the referral for an audiological evaluation of hearing loss occurs prior to any interaction with the child that might make the parent suspect that the child is not accessing information in the environment through audition or is partially accessing auditory information.

Thus, a serious concern about universal newborn hearing screening programs is that such an early age of identification of hearing loss could have a potentially negative impact on bonding and interaction between parent and child due to grieving. A negative outcome could easily result without appropriate intervention services and in the absence of specific counseling skills of the provider. In order to address this serious concern, the Colorado Home Intervention Program (CHIP) established a system that provides immediate contact with a trained professional, the Co-Hear Coordinator. This contact occurs almost simultaneously with the time a parent receives information about a diagnosis of hearing loss in the child. This professional is probably not the individual who will eventually provide ongoing services for the family, but will remain with the family until a choice about intervention programs is made.

Several very important issues must be addressed in universal newborn hearing screening programs. Even mothers whose children are not diagnosed with a hearing disability might experience postpartum depression. Since hormonal changes may be extreme following delivery, appropriate support for families is essential. The Colorado Home Intervention Program has designed a follow-through program that provides families with the power and responsibility for making choices appropriate to their family, such as how quickly they wish to schedule a re-screen appointment. The family is offered the opportunity to have a professional visit in their home to provide additional information and answer any questions the family might have. Diagnosing audiologists throughout the state provide families with a resource manual describing services available either in their geographic area or throughout the state. Counseling on communication methods is not provided at the time of diagnosis of the hearing loss, but through the Co-Hear Coordinator. The families determine how quickly they wish to have information provided and what kind of information they want. Some families make decisions rapidly about what communication method they wish to learn, although others opt for a much longer time to make the decision.

Parent-infant facilitators have received training in the following counseling aspects: (1) discussing difficult issues; (2) providing a diagnosis; (3) listening techniques; (4) family systems; (5) cultural competence; (6) making difficult referrals; (7) providing objective, un-biased information; (8) counseling strategies appropriate for families in grieving with anger, depression, or guilt; (9) making decisions concerning when to facilitate, when to provide guidance, or when to instruct; and (10) establishing trust relationships with families.

Even if professionals did know exactly what needed to be done by each family from the time of diagnosis of the hearing loss, this knowledge would be useless unless families could be convinced that such a plan of action needed to be adopted. The problem becomes even more complex because research is not substantial enough to provide answers for all the questions posed by these families.

THE GRIEVING PROCESS

Pianta and Marvin (1992) developed the Reaction to Diagnosis Intervention (RDI), which probes for episodic recall of events and experiences that occurred at the time of diagnosis. Parents are asked to relate their emotions associated with that experience, the change in these emotions since the time of diagnosis, and their search for reasons for this experience. Families with resolved grieving report changes in their emotions since the diagnosis of the hearing loss. They indicate that they are able to move on in life and have suspended the search for a reason. Families with resolved grieving are able to provide accurate representations of their child's abilities and provide balanced statements regarding the benefits to self. The resolution of grief can be evidenced through feelings, actions, or thoughts.

Families with unresolved grieving indicate one or several of the following characteristics: (1) emotionally overwhelmed; (2) angrily preoccupied; (3) neutralizing their emotions; (4) feelings of depression or passivity; (5) cognitive distortions including unrealistic beliefs, denial, or pursuit of wished-for realities such as a different diagnosis; and (6) disorganization or confusion. Families with unresolved grieving actively search for reasons. In these cases, attention to the reality of the child's needs is displaced by the need to find a reason. This need for a reason is often so strong that it distracts parents from attending to painful emotions. The search for a reason often continues even when told repeatedly by professionals that no reason will be found and that cause will not change the diagnosis or prognosis. Families who are unable to resolve their grief may be stuck in the past or cut-off from the experience of the diagnosis, indicating no emotion at the time. Their story about the diagnosis may be confused and disorganized making it difficult to understand. Emotionally overwhelmed families have strong expressions of sadness and/or pain. There is an enlistment of sympathy and a feeling that the crisis continues in the present. Families who are angrily preoccupied express active and thematic anger and enlist endorsement of this anger from the professional. Families who have neutralized their emotions report no perception of negative emotion associated with the diagnosis. Some families have clear distortion of the expectations regarding their child's condition and future. They may express unbalanced perceptions regarding the benefits versus the negative aspects of the experience, either idealizing the experience or painting a picture of no hope. Families may express confusion or incoherence through contradictions in content of their stories about their experiences. Some families lose their train of thought and need to be re-oriented by the professional. They may ramble or oscillate between polarized perceptions, i.e., all good or all bad, all painful or all beneficial.

In a pilot study of 16 families conducted by Siegel (2000), there was a strong trend toward a significant finding based upon the age of identification. Of these 16 families, 10 had resolved their grieving, while 6 had not. The average age of identification for the resolved group was 8.1 months and for the unresolved group was 16 months of age. The interview was conducted at a mean of 37.72 months since the identification of hearing loss for the resolved group and 39 months since the identification of hearing loss for the unresolved group. No differences by caregiver education, gender, or degree of hearing loss were evident. The families who had resolved their grieving had children with expressive language skills that were 6 months better than the families with unresolved grieving.

Although there is a need for significantly more research data, there is a strong indication that resolution of grief may be highly related to language development of the child. Other studies indicate a strong relationship between maternal bonding and language development. It is reasonable to hypothesize that appropriate counseling skills of providers can improve maternal-child interaction, which can then have a better impact on language development and a quicker resolution of parental grieving. Because these studies are not studies of causal relationships, it is also possible that improved techniques that will facilitate better language development could improve maternal bonding and resolution of grief, or that counseling strategies to help parents resolve grief could create better maternal bonding and better language development of the child. In any of these scenarios, emphasis upon improved counseling skills is warranted.

PARENTAL STRESS

In addition to parental grieving, parental stress has been identified as a significant factor for families with children who have hearing loss. Abidin (1995) differentiated three different types of parenting stress: (1) maternal characteristics known to affect parenting ability, such as depression or lack of social support; (2) child characteristics, such as a difficult temperament that might include learned patterns of defiance, non-compliance, or demanding behavior; and (3) difficulties in interacting with the child, such as the parent feeling rejected, abused by, or disappointed in the child, which is a result of the parent-child bond either being threatened or not adequately established.

In a study of 184 hearing mothers of children with hearing loss (Siegel, Sedey, and Yoshinaga-Itano in press), parental stress was measured through the short form of the Parental Stress Index (PSI; Abidin 1995). The Parenting Events Scale (Crnic and Greenberg 1990) consists of twenty statements about daily routines (i.e., being nagged, whined at, complained to, or having difficulty getting privacy). Parents are asked to rate the frequency of the occurrence on a 4-point scale and the degree to which the behavior is a "big hassle" or "no hassle." The responses on this scale were highly related to the Parental Stress Inventory. The Family Support Scale (Dunst, Jenkins, and Trivette 1984) consists of 18 sources of family support (parents, friends, spouse, etc.). Families rate the availability of the source of support and whether the support is helpful.

Parental distress on the PSI increases as the intensity of hassles on the Parenting Events Scale increases, and the amount of social support decreases. When daily routines are rated as "big hassle," parents obtained higher stress ratings on all three stress subscales. When parents report that they lack sources of social support from family, friends, spouse, or agencies and report lower income, they also experience higher degrees of parental stress. Increased stress in parent-child interactions occurs with disabilities in addition to hearing loss, more delayed language relative to chronological age and less severe degrees of hearing loss. When all variables were controlled for, the child's ethnicity, age of identification, mode of communication used, months between age of identification and child's age at the time of observation, and maternal education did not predict maternal stress on any of the three subscales.

The degree of parental stress reported by these mothers was similar to the findings of Meadow-Orlans (1997). Parents of children with hearing loss experience stress at similar levels to parents of children with cerebral palsy (Siegel, Sedey, and Yoshinaga-Itano in press). Development of counseling strategies that will assist providers in decreasing parental stress should be a focus for training of early intervention providers.

Emotional Availability

Maternal bonding was evaluated through the Emotional Availability Scales developed by Biringen, Robinson, and Emde (1993). This scale evaluates maternal dimensions, child dimensions, and reciprocity in the relationship. Maternal dimensions include maternal sensitivity, maternal structuring/intrusiveness, and maternal frustration/hostility. Child dimensions include child sensitivity, child's responsiveness to his or her mother, child's involvement with his or her mother, and child's frustration/hostility towards his or her mother.

Maternal sensitivity involves warmth and emotional connectivity to the child. Optimal sensitivity indicates positive, appropriate, and creative emotional communication with the child. Mothers with maternal sensitivity show genuine, authentic, and congruent interest, pleasure, and amusement. Optimal sensitivity is characterized by warm smiles, interested eye contact, comforting and playful physical contact, pleasant facial expressions, and tone of voice. The maternal behaviors are rhythmic, timely, flexible, and adaptable to the demands or needs of the child.

Maternal structuring and intrusiveness involves the ability of the mother to follow the child's lead during play, to set limits for appropriate behavior or misbehavior, and to provide a supportive frame within the context of allowing the child to maximize his or her autonomy. Child responsiveness is reflected in the child's eagerness or willingness to be engaged with his or her mother following her suggestion or bid for exchange. Child responsiveness includes a display of clear signs of pleasure in the interaction. The degree to which the child attends to and is engaged with his or her mother in play, the balance between the child's autonomy in play and the need to draw the mother into play, are components of child responsiveness.

Maternal sensitivity predicted significant and positive expressive language gain (Pressman et al. 2000). The more emotionally connected the mother was to the child, the greater the expressive language gain of the child when measured at two different ages. Strategies for teaching parents skills in improving emotional availability have had success with other populations of at-risk children. An emphasis in counseling skills to improve sensitivity, scaffolding, and ability to deal with frustration in interactions would be beneficial for early intervention providers working with families of young deaf and hard-of-hearing infants and toddlers.

PERSONAL-SOCIAL DEVELOPMENT

The Minnesota Child Development Inventory includes a sub-test that measures personal-social development (Ireton and Thwing 1972). These measures include social skills, and emotional and behavioral development. Many, but not all of these items, are language dependent. Over 70% of the variance in personal-social skill development is accounted for by the symbolic play development, expressive language development, and degree of hearing loss of the child.

Children identified early had better personal-social quotients in the first three years of life than children identified later. The age of identification effect was found by gender, by degree of hearing loss category, by mode of communication, and at each testing age. Symbolic play and expressive language do not account for all of the variance in personal-social development. Degree of hearing loss also contributes information. Interestingly, parents report that children with mild hearing loss have poorer personal-social skill development than children with moderate to profound hearing loss when they are identified later, even when they have strong language skills. Thus, the relationship of early identification/intervention to personal-social skill development is the strongest for children with mild hearing loss.

Some have argued that children with mild hearing loss do not demonstrate significant enough developmental delay to warrant newborn hearing screening. The personal-social skill difference appears to counter this argument. An implication for intervention for children identified later is that a much greater emphasis needs to be placed upon remediation of delays in this developmental area.

Development of Self

Studies of the development of self-concept in early childhood have focused on self-recognition (Lewis and Brooks-Gunn 1979), self-evaluation (Stipek 1983), or self-regulation (Kopp 1982). Stipek, Gralinski, and Kopp (1990) developed a parent-report questionnaire about self-concept development. Self description/evaluation and self-regulation are two factors examined through this Self-Concept Questionnaire. Pressman (2000), in a study on the early self-development of children with hearing loss, found that both self-recognition and self-description/evaluation developed with age between 14 and 40 months of age. Deaf and hard-of-hearing children always passed the self-recognition items prior to the self-description/evaluation items, similar to the development of children with normal hearing. Self-recognition scores increased significantly from 14 to 40 months when children were deaf or hard of hearing. The linear development between self-recognition and age was completely mediated by expressive language. Self-description/evaluation also increased significantly with age and decreased significantly as the age at which hearing loss was identified increased, even when child and family characteristics were controlled. Expressive language partially, but not completely, mediated the relation between self-description/evaluation and both age and age of identification. Age of identification, even beyond the effects of improvement of language had a significant relationship with the development of self.

Thus, the development of self, possibly the development of strong self-esteem and self-concept have both a language and social-emotional and/or non-verbal component. Language development, as found with other aspects of social-emotional development, is highly related to the development of self.

EMOTIONAL RESPONSE TO THE REFERRAL FOR FOLLOW-UP TESTING

Abdala de Uzcategui (1997) conducted a study of parents referred from two different hospital newborn screening programs. Hospital #1 was a suburban hospital with approximately 1600 births per year with a referral rate at hospital discharge of 4%. Hospital screening was done by both volunteers and audiologists. The socio-economic status of the patient population in Hospital #1 was predominantly middle income. One-hundred surveys were sent to all families referred for follow-through between April 1995 and April 1996. Fifty-five percent of the families returned these surveys. Of these, five had children with confirmed hearing loss. The results from the families with confirmed hearing loss are included in the parental responses. Hospital #2 was an urban inner-city hospital with approximately 1600 births from November 1995 to November 1996. The socio-economic status of the patient population in Hospital #2 ranged from lower to middle income with the vast majority of the patients being recipients of Medicaid. Screening and results were provided by audiologists. One-hundred-one surveys were mailed with an overall 22% return rate. The referral rate at hospital discharge was 10% for this hospital. No confirmed hearing losses were reported during this time period. The survey instrument had 46 questions and was a Likert-type questionnaire with a 1 to 4 scale response designed by Eiserman (1997). Some of the items to which the parents responded by rating themselves were:

Confused (didn't understand what the results really meant);
Informed (I understood the results and need for another test);
Angry (that this was happening to me and my child);
Calm (not worried about it at that point);

Afraid (about the unknown challenges of a child with a hearing loss);
Comforted (by staff who helped me to be hopeful);
Depressed (about what would be lost if my child had a hearing loss)
Encouraged (that I could handle it if my child had a hearing loss);
Certain (convinced that my child did, in fact, have a hearing loss);
Doubtful (not convinced that my child has a hearing loss);
Impatient (wanting more conclusive results sooner);
Patient (willing to just wait and see before reacting);
Frustrated (by lack of information and/or conflicting information);
Satisfied (with how my concerns and questions were addressed);
Shocked (didn't know what I felt—almost numb of feelings);
Sad (about what my child would be facing in life);
Guilty (feeling like my child's condition was my fault);
Blame (feeling that someone did something wrong to cause this);
Lonely (feeling that no one understood what I was feeling); or
Accepting (willing to accept the fact of a hearing loss if necessary).

Some additional questions included: What did you understand to be the results of your child's first hearing test? Did the results of the first hearing test make you more aware of your child's hearing? Since the first hearing test have you had your child's hearing tested again? Was a hearing loss identified as a result of the hearing test? Have you found yourself paying attention to how your child hears different sounds? How much thought did you give to the language development of a child with a hearing loss?

The findings from this survey indicate that most of the parents who are referred for additional audiological testing do not express significant emotional harm. (A few results of this survey are included in table I, figures 1, 2, and 3). This study did not include a control group of families who passed the universal newborn hearing screening. Tharpe (1999) reported that there were no significant differences between the parental stress and parental depression of parents whose infants passed the newborn hearing screening and those parents whose infants were referred for additional testing.

The results of these surveys can assist the provider in understanding how parents respond to information about the hearing screening results. This information should provide valuable insight into the most effective means of conveying information to the parents. Parents indicated that they wanted to have some decision about the timing of the re-screening. Some parents preferred to have their child re-screened the following day, while others were content to wait for a

Table I

Question	Not at all	Not Much	Some-what	A lot	No Response
Shocked (didn't know what I felt-almost numb of feeling)	N = 33 47.8%	N = 17 24.6%	N = 12 17.4%	N = 5 7.3%	N = 2 2.9%
Depressed (About what would be lost if my child had a hearing loss)	N = 30 43.5%	N = 14 20.3%	N = 12 17.4%	N = 8 11.6%	N = 5 7.2%
Informed (I understood the results and need for another test)	N = 40 58%	N = 16 23.2%	N = 2 2.9%	N = 6 8.7%	N = 5 7.2%

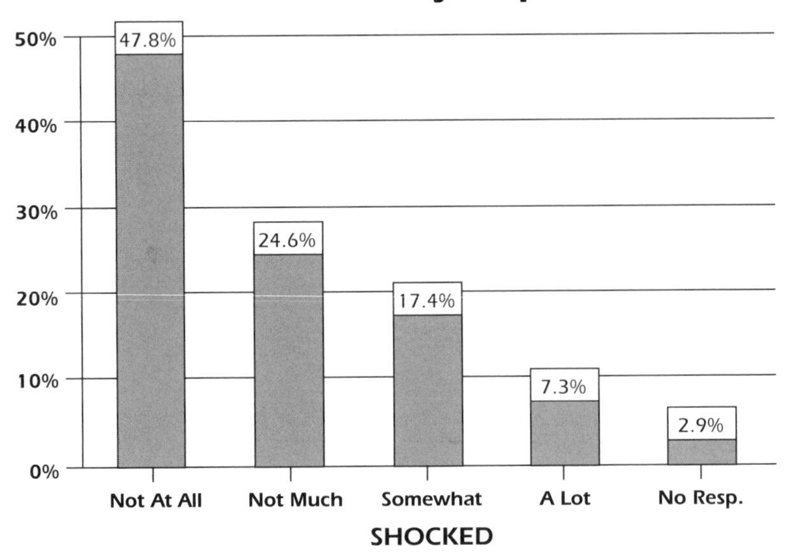

Figure 1. Parent survey responses from parents referred for additional testing prior to hospital discharge regarding their feelings of shock.

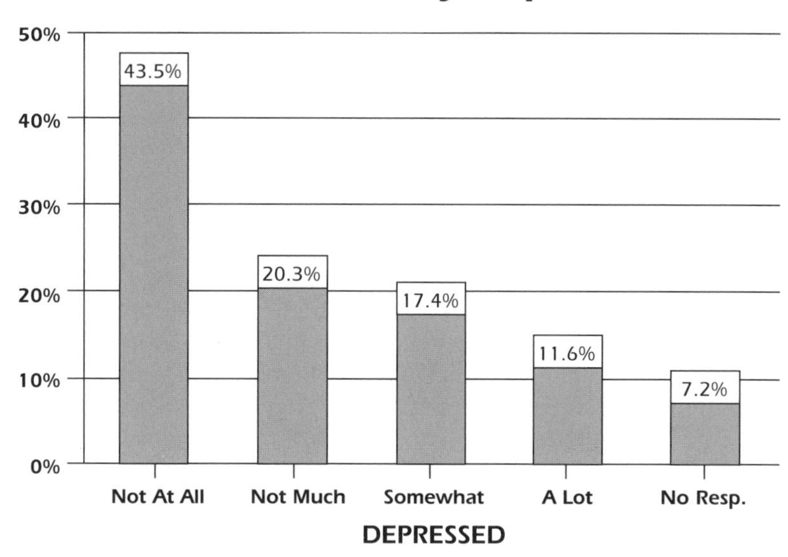

Figure 2. Parent survey responses from families referred for additional testing prior to hospital discharge regarding their feelings of depression.

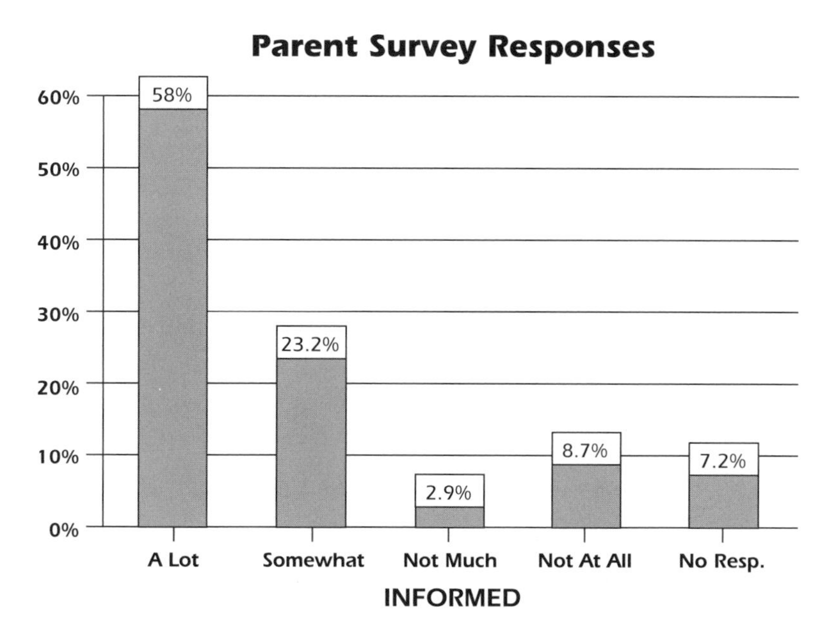

Figure 3. Parent survey responses from families referred for additional testing prior to hospital discharge regarding how informed they felt.

few weeks or several days before returning. Valuable information was obtained from the survey. Parents provided important information about what aspects of the screening program and referral for additional hearing testing needed to be improved and gave suggestions about how these improvements could be implemented.

SUMMARY

Early identification of hearing loss in conjunction with early intervention is associated with improved social-emotional development. More highly developed personal-social development, development of self, reduction in parental stress, improved emotional availability in the maternal-child interaction, and resolution of grieving appear to be highly related to language development. A significant relationship between language development and early identification/intervention has been previously reported (Yoshinaga-Itano et al. 1998). Regardless of the directionality of causality, there is strong indication that significant emphasis should be placed upon improved counseling techniques to address these specific aspects of social-emotional characteristics.

REFERENCES

Abdala de Uzcategui, C. 1997. Refer rate and parental anxiety in newborn hearing screening in the state of Colorado. Unpublished doctoral dissertation. Boulder, CO: University of Colorado.

Abidin, R. R. 1995. *Parental Stress Index*, 3rd Edition. Odessa, FL: Psychological Assessment Resources.

Apuzzo, M., and Yoshinaga-Itano, C. 1995. Early identification of infants with significant hearing loss and the Minnesota Child Development Inventory. *Seminars in Hearing* 16(2):124–39.

Biringen, Z., Robinson, J. L., and Emde, R. N. 1993. Manual for scoring the emotional availability scales: Infancy to early childhood version. Unpublished manuscript. Denver, CO: University of Colorado Health Sciences Center.

Crnic, K. A. and Greenberg, M. T. 1990. Minor parenting stress with young children. *Child Development* 61:1628–37.

Dunst, C. J., Jenkins, V., and Trivette, C. M. 1984. The Family Support Scale: Reliability and Validity. *Journal of Individual, Family, and Community Wellness* 1:45–52.

Eiserman, W. 1996. Parent survey. Unpublished survey. Boulder, CO: University of Colorado.

Ireton, H. and Thwing, E. 1972. *The Minnesota Child Development Inventory.* University of Minnesota, Minneapolis, MN.

Kopp, C. B. 1982. Antecedents of self-regulation: A developmental perspective. *Developmental Psychology* 26:199–214.

Lewis, M. and Brooks-Gunn, J. 1979. *Social Cognition and the Acquisition of Self.* New York: Plenum Press.

Luterman, D. 1987. *Deafness in the Family*. Boston: Little Brown.
Luterman, D. 1995. *Counseling Persons with Communication Disorders and Their Families*. Austin, TX: PRO-ED.
Luterman, D., Kurtzer-White, E. and Seewald, R. C. 1999. *The Young Deaf Child*. Timonium, MD: York Press.
Meadow-Orlans, K. 1997. Effect of mother and infant hearing status on interactions at twelve and eighteen months. *Journal of Deaf Studies and Deaf Education* 2:26–36.
Obenchain, P., Menn, L., and Yoshinaga-Itano, C. 2000. Can speech development at thirty-six months in children with hearing loss be predicted from information available in the second year of life? In *Language, Speech and Social-Emotional Development of Children Who Are Deaf and Hard-of-Hearing: The Early Years*, eds. C. Yoshinaga-Itano and A. Sedey. The Volta Review 100(5).
Pressman, L. 2000. Early self-development in children with hearing loss. Unpublished doctoral dissertation. Boulder, CO: University of Colorado.
Pressman, L., Pipp-Siegel, S., Yoshinaga-Itano, C., and Deas, A. M. 1999. Maternal sensitivity predicts language gain in preschool children who are deaf and hard of hearing. In *Language, Speech and Social-Emotional Development of Children Who Are Deaf and Hard of Hearing: The Early Years*, eds. C. Yoshinaga-Itano and A. Sedey. The Volta Review 100(5).
Pressman, L., Pipp-Siegel, S., Yoshinaga-Itano, C., Kubicek, L., and Emde, R. N. 2000. A comparison of the links between emotional availability and language gain in young children with and without hearing loss. In *Language, Speech and Social-Emotional Development of Children Who Are Deaf and Hard-of-Hearing: The Early Years*, eds. C. Yoshinaga-Itano and A. Sedey. The Volta Review 100(5).
Siegel, S. 2000. Resolution of grief of parents with young children with hearing loss. Unpublished manuscript. Boulder, CO: University of Colorado.
Siegel, S., Sedey, A., and Yoshinaga-Itano, C. in press. Parental stress of hearing mothers of young children with hearing loss. *Journal of Deaf Studies and Deaf Education.*
Stipek, D. 1983. A developmental analysis of pride and shame. *Human Development* 26:42–54.
Stipek, D. J., Gralinski, H. and Kopp, C. B. 1990. Self-concept development in the toddler years. *Developmental Psychology* 26:972–7.
Tharpe, A. 1999. Early identification of hearing loss in children: Ethical and legal issues associated with newborn hearing screening. ASHA Annual Convention (November 18–21, 1999), San Francisco, CA.
Wallace, V., Menn, L., and Yoshinaga-Itano, C. 2000. Is babble the gateway to speech for all children?: A longitudinal study of children who are deaf and hard-of-hearing. In *Language, Speech and Social-Emotional Development of Children Who Are Deaf and Hard-of-Hearing: The Early Years*, eds. C. Yoshinaga-Itano and A. Sedey. The Volta Review 100(5).
Yoshinaga-Itano, C., and Apuzzo, M. 1998a. Identification of hearing loss after 18 months is not early enough. *American Annals of the Deaf* 143:380–7.
Yoshinaga-Itano, C., and Apuzzo, M. 1998b. The development of deaf and hard-of-hearing children identified early through the high risk registry. *American Annals of the Deaf* 143:416–4.
Yoshinaga-Itano, C., Coulter, D., and Thomson, V. 2000. Infant hearing impairment and universal hearing screening. *Journal of Perinatology* 20(8): 132–37.
Yoshinaga-Itano, C., Coulter, D., and Thomson, V. in press. Developmental outcomes of children born in Colorado hospitals with universal newborn

hearing screening programs. Newton, V. ed., Disorders of the Special Senses. *Seminars in Neonatology.*

Yoshinaga-Itano, C., and Sedey, A. 2000. Early speech development of children who are deaf and hard-of-hearing: Interrelationships with language and hearing. In *Language, Speech and Social-Emotional Development of Children Who Are Deaf and Hard-of-Hearing: The Early Years,* eds. C. Yoshinaga-Itano and A. Sedey. The Volta Revew 100(5).

Yoshinaga-Itano, C., Sedey, A., Coulter, D., and Mehl, A. 1998. Language of early- and later-identified children with hearing loss. *Pediatrics* 102(5): 1161–71.

Chapter ▪ 3

After Screening . . . The Diagnostic Process

Marilyn W. Neault

> To know that we know what we know,
> and that we do not know what we do not know,
> that is true knowledge.
> - Thoreau (after Confucius)

I feel privileged to have worked for almost two decades in the same town as Dr. Luterman's Thayer-Lindsley Nursery program for families of deaf and hard of hearing children. Because of Dr. Luterman's ambivalence about newborn hearing screening, it is ironic that he has been preparing for the aftermath of screening—and preparing us for it—for over three decades. The Thayer-Lindsley Nursery program is a safe place for parents to be when they have a baby newly diagnosed as deaf or hard of hearing. They want to get started on a habilitative path, but they are just beginning to learn their options for their child's communication and education. The parents of a two-month-old baby should not yet choose whether they want voice-off American Sign Language (ASL), sign-supported English, Signing Exact English, Cued Speech, auditory-oral, auditory-verbal, or any other single method for communicating with their child. They need time to think about their own priorities for their child and what might work for their family, while their child's communicative style unfolds. They need to share their questions, hopes, dreams, and confusions with other parents. Taking time to learn does not mean that the parents of a two-month-old should delay natural parent-child communication, hearing aid fitting, and visits with an early intervention "coach" to support, reassure, and train them while they are learning their options.

Some early intervention programs for babies who are deaf, while being excellent programs, are highly methodology-specific, and not places to learn about choices. Those choices should take place in an unpressured, non-biased, and nonjudgmental milieu.

I am fortunate to work in a fine children's hospital, a teaching hospital of Harvard Medical School, with a terrific group of audiologists. Our Department of Otolaryngology and Communication Disorders is large, with nine pediatric otolaryngologists plus fellows and residents, several speech-language pathologists, the Communication Enhancement Center which includes speech, occupational therapy, and software development for nonspeaking and nonwriting individuals, and our Boston Center for Deaf and Hard of Hearing Children which combines psychology, psychiatry, speech and language, developmental pediatrics, and other specialities to assess and help with the complexities that deaf children and their families experience. We have a dozen audiologists at the hospital site and seven others at two satellite locations, and we provide over 11,000 audiology visits for children per year. The opportunity to learn from the parents of so many children is a formidable one. Our audiology and otolaryngology floor at the hospital is a busy place, with a waiting room full of active, napless toddlers with ear infections whose tired parents don't realize why they are speaking loudly to their children. In this busy context, we need to preserve quiet moments to connect with and listen to families.

TIMES HAVE CHANGED

Times have changed for babies who are deaf or hard of hearing. Earlier diagnosis means earlier access to language. Many of these babies who were identified at birth have normal-range language skills at the age when toddlers with no language used to be identified as being deaf. Whatever difficulties the audiologists, teachers, and parents encounter because of the early diagnosis, the outcomes are so good that we should make the road leading to those outcomes smoother rather than go back to the old way.

Times have changed for the audiologist. We meet the babies so young that the first test looks for a physiological response rather than a behavioral one. A single appointment may involve several technology-dependent measures. Soon to be gone, thankfully, are the days when many deaf children came in for their first test when they were old enough to do separate-ear audiograms by conditioned play audiometry, so that auditory brainstem response (ABR) evaluation was not needed. Gone are the days when a threshold ABR was finished when the audiologist saw a flat line in response to alternating polarity clicks at the intensity limits of the stimulus generator. Now a single appointment for a deaf or hard of hearing infant may involve separate ABR recordings for rarefaction and condensation clicks to check for a cochlear microphonic response, frequency-specific ABR thresholds, otoacoustic emissions, multifrequency tympanometry, and even real-ear-to-coupler difference measures if the baby already has earmolds. This increase in test procedures takes place in an era of demands for audiologists to see more and more patients to compensate for decreased reimbursement to the hospital from health plans. It is tempting to fall into a model of care in which the test results are the finish line, not the starting gate.

Preserving space, time, and mood for the more important aspects of helpfulness is a challenge in today's health care environment. On our staff, when we realize that one of the audiologists is in the midst of a new diagnosis, the others close ranks and pick up the other duties she might have, to allow her time to spend with the new family. Scheduling for such an eventuality beforehand is next to impossible, because we cannot diagnose children over the phone to know how to schedule them; if we could do that, they would not need to see us.

Test proliferation brings the challenge of continuing education and credentialing. An audiologist, even after twenty years of experience in the field, should not be performing a new test without theoretical grounding, training, and mentoring in its use. For audiologists to keep up to speed on a growing number of procedures is daunting.

For many years, it has been a consistent finding that 50% of deaf and hard of hearing children have no known etiology for their hearing status. That 50% is shrinking rapidly, thanks in large part to three factors: (1) improved imaging of the cochlea to find subtle dysplasia; (2) cytomegalovirus (CMV); screens in the first weeks of life to detect otherwise asymptomatic CMV in babies with hearing loss; and (3) genetic testing for the connexin 26 mutation, the most common cause of nonsyndromic recessive sensorineural hearing loss. Diagnosis of hearing loss no longer consists of an audiogram plus a quick peek in the ears by an otolaryngologist who signs a medical clearance form for the sale of a hearing aid. Now the audiologist, otolaryngologist, geneticist, radiologist, infectious disease specialist, and neurologist are getting to know one another quite well in the diagnostic process.

For parents, the "diagnostic process" must seem like a series of administrative hoops through which they must jump. Securing the referral from the pediatrician, the authorization number from the health plan, the appointment, the time off from work, the arrangements for the sibling coming home from school, parking, outpatient registration, and, at long last, the crowded elevator to . . . yet another desk to check in . . .

Times have changed for the health care system aspects of infant hearing. The "up" note is that outpatient diagnostic audiological evaluations now occur for the correct babies (those who have not passed a newborn hearing screening test). Gone are the days when parents would have to bring a van and a third adult with their triplet premies for initial diagnostic ABR evaluations, scheduled for two hours and over $200 each. Now, at least two or perhaps all three babies will have passed a newborn hearing screening test prior to hospital discharge, and will have been properly and efficiently served. Universal newborn hearing screening does create other "system" problems, however. The cost of the in-hospital hearing screening tests are poorly reimbursed, particularly by health plans that pay a single package price for a newborn admission. Diagnostically, the work up for hearing loss in newborns requires interdisciplinary efforts, with plenty of un-reimbursed time spent in communication among professionals and in trying to set up appointments in a family-friendly way. Communication with the baby's "medical home" (usually the primary care provider's office) is crucial, so that the primary care physician, who may have known and will know the family for years, can help to orchestrate and support their care (American Academy of Pediatrics 1992). In fact, after the diagnosis and with the parents' permission, the audiologist should call the primary care physician before the family does, so that the physician can support and guide them. Given the family's potential stress and distress, and given the potentially good experience for the family and good outcome for the baby if the diagnostic process goes well, the extra time and effort are never to be regretted.

Times have changed for early intervention programs. They are experiencing a three- to four-fold increase in the numbers of children under the age of three years enrolled because of their hearing status. Therefore, the need to train more providers of specialized early intervention for deaf and hard of hearing babies is pressing. There are not more children needing services; they simply enter early intervention before age six months rather than a year or two later. Many of the babies who used to be detected "late" have mild and moderate hearing losses. Early intervention providers may not know quite what to do with babies who turn their heads toward their spoken names and appear to meet their early auditory milestones, and so training is needed in steps to avoid the subtle but pervasive effects of mild-moderate hearing loss on language and socialization. Early intervention providers also must learn about cochlear implants, because some parents are making decisions about implantation at the same time that they are learning about communication options for their infant. The cochlear implant decision is becoming far more closely tied to the choice of communication modalities than hearing aid fitting ever has been.

A growing challenge for specialized programs for deaf and hard of hearing infants is the need to continue to look at the development of the whole child. Thirty percent of these babies have other developmental challenges, many of which will not yet have surfaced upon enrollment. It is no longer safe nor helpful to say, with any confidence, to parents that hearing loss is their baby's only challenge and that she or he sparkles in all other areas, when the baby is two-months-old. Seizure disorder might become evident in another month, or autism in another year or two.

Another challenge for the early intervention system is to provide more modality-neutral entry points for parents of deaf and hard of hearing infants, with providers who are not only trained in, but actually supportive of, a variety of methods. Many superlative parent-infant programs do what they do extremely well, be it an oral or a bilingual-bi-cultural method. Providers should trust parents' self-knowledge about the way they will be able to do the best parenting and language nurturing with their own child, provided that the parents are familiar with the options. Unfortunately, the passion and commitment required to implement some methods do not allow for parental exploration of their own priorities and of other options, during a time when they are just beginning to observe their own baby's communicative style. Parents may feel too guilty to tell their single-method provider that they want to look into another mode of communication or another program option. Because the baby's hearing loss may have been identified before other developmental challenges emerge, and because the baby's innate ability to make best progress in a given modality may not be evident early, both the parents and the early intervention provider need to support the notion of changing course or adding new tools if the child's language is not flourishing at developmental check points.

Times have changed more for the parents than for anyone else in the child-hearing domain. Parents are being told that their child is deaf or hard of hearing before they have had a chance to suspect it. Prior to universal newborn screening, parents would suspect hearing loss, ask the pediatrician about it, secure a referral, call for an appointment, and go to the audiology clinic. The diagnosis, even if devastating, often imparted a little relief, because the parents were validated in their observations of their own child and because they now had a concrete diagnosis with which to work. Now the diagnosis "happens to" parents, in answer to a question they have not yet asked. It happens at a time when they are asked to trust wiggly lines on a computer screen instead of observations that the child does not turn his head nor speak. It happens when they are sleep-deprived. It happens when they are still learning how to feed and diaper the baby. It happens at a time of intense contact and scrutiny from relatives and friends, as new babies seem to be as publicly owned as pregnancies. The parents may not have much opportunity to cry, argue, bang pans, and support each other spontaneously in their own way and in the privacy they deserve. Finding out that one's child has a permanent hearing impairment is not a bed of roses at any age, but, while best for the baby, diagnosis during the newborn period has thorns in different places.

Even the experience of parents whose babies had a "false positive" result on a newborn hearing screening test is thorny. A nurse, technician, or a piece of paper that notifies the parent of the "refer" status may fail to explain the screening process and the statistics involved enough to help them understand that the referral is not a diagnosis. During the time between the referral and the diagnostic test, the parents may feel frantic. Afterward, if the baby's hearing proves to be normal, the parents may still be waiting for the "other shoe to drop," and they may feel that the child's hearing is vulnerable in some way. Providing information about a screening process, rather than imparting only the results, reduces the parents' long-term concerns about the child. For newborn hearing screening, explaining the process to parents includes informing them in the pre-admission maternity packet that the screening will happen; explaining that of every 1,000 babies screened, as many as 30 will not pass the first screening, but 26 of those 30 children will turn out to have entirely normal hearing. Thanking the parents most sincerely for participating in a process that helps deaf babies enormously is important. A father of a baby who was a "bilateral refer" on a newborn hearing screening test told me that he wished fervently that he had been told that a "bilateral refer" was more likely to be the "real thing" than a unilateral refer, because he would have taken off from work to be with his wife and feel part of the process when she was told that their beautiful baby daughter is deaf.

THE DIAGNOSTIC PROCESS

The diagnostic process has more steps and may be revisited more often than it was a decade or two ago. The change in the information volunteered by parents during case histories reveals this evolution, past and (speculatively) future:

1970: "His doctor said that if he's not talking by the time he's two, we'd test his hearing."

1980: "He doesn't react to the microwave beeping when his food is warmed up, and I remember his sister doing that."

1988: "We tried five behavioral audiograms and finally went for an ABR."

1995: "Her CT scan was normal in 1985, but when her hearing got even worse, we had it done again before her cochlear implant and this time they found the enlarged vestibular aqueducts." (CT scans give more fine-grained images now, so that previously "normal" cochleas may be found to have subtle malformations found with hearing loss.)

1998: "I remember his big sister used to hear my cell phone ring inside the diaper bag when we were out shopping, but he never notices it."

2000: "After his big brother's hearing loss was picked up by newborn screening, we got tested, and I carry one kind of connexin 26 mutation and my husband carries a different kind."

2003: "When he was in the NICU for such a long time, they switched his antibiotic because they found he had that A1555G mutation" (the mitochondrial mutation associated with sensitivity to the ototoxic effects of aminoglycoside antibiotics) "and they didn't want him to lose his hearing from the drugs."

2005: "We had the genetic testing before he was born, and he was positive for PAX 3 on chromosome 2 [a gene location identified for Waardenburg Syndrome], just like my aunt who is deaf, so we started taking sign language classes when I was five months pregnant. Now that he's off to such a good start, he'll get his first cochlear implant next week and then if all goes well he'll get the other one in two months. He'll be in the clinical trial for neurotrophins to preserve the nerve cells because it might help the implant work better."

While following cues provided by the parents, the audiologist engages in the process of diagnosis, that of formulating hypotheses about the nature or cause of a condition, and systematically ruling them out. Although the audiologist cannot make a diagnosis in the medical sense, the diagnosis of the degree and type of hearing loss most certainly arises from the audiological battery.

The word diagnosis arises from the Greek root meaning "through knowing." It is through knowing that parents can move forward, not through information. Information is everywhere, too much of it. We scan it, sift it, and weigh it. Only when information is understood, and melds with some internal perception, can it generate knowledge, which in turn can affect beliefs and actions. Involvement of the parent or parents in the diagnostic process to the greatest extent possible helps them to sift information so that it may generate knowledge.

What may help parents feel valued and participatory in the diagnostic process? What may help them to get "back in the driver's seat?" First, it helps to let parents know what will happen during the session. Will there be a chance to talk before and after the tests? What tests will be administered, and what do they assess? Second, it helps to make a little "small talk" before the tests begin. Questions asked after the test results are delivered seem overly loaded with prognostic significance, so it helps to learn a little about the family's situation before starting. "Is this delightful baby your first child?" "Are you planning to work outside the home?" "What kind of work do you do?" "Are you having any luck with day care arrangements?" "Do you have relatives in the area?" If you find out that the baby's mother is starting a new full-time job next Monday, having this situation in mind can help to explain the mother's distress over the schedule when follow-up appointments are established after the test. Remembering who the family members are and how to say their names helps convey caring.

In explaining test results, matching the parents' speaking patterns to some extent may help their understanding of the results. A parent who speaks in short, simple words and sentences, with many pauses, may process information best when it is delivered at that same pace, whether or not she has presented herself as an "internet warrior." A parent who is comfortable using polysyllabic medical terminology may appreciate an explanation laced with such terms. Finding out the parents' past experiences with people who are deaf or hard of hearing also helps immensely in understanding their reaction to the news that their baby has a hearing loss.

A true listening attitude on the part of the audiologist includes pauses that are as long as they need to be for the parents to begin to react, but does not include subtle behaviors that convey "hurry" such as glancing at the watch or uncrossing the legs as if to stand up and end the session. It behooves the audiologist to let the explanation of the diagnosis go in the direction of the parent's first question, rather than to continue on the audiologist's pre-set agenda for what seems important for the parents to hear. They may not hear much after learning the diagnosis, but might prefer to go home, feel safe, and come back another day to learn more. At follow-up visits, parents may come in asking about a possible diagnosis or intervention about which they have learned from an acquaintance or on the internet. The relevance of their discovery must be discussed, because they may be very attached to an intervention they have discovered themselves, as a healthy way of regaining control after being given a diagnosis which they did not seek.

Often a parent may feel "stuck" and unable to hear and understand more than the basic label applied to the test results. The audiologist may feel that the parents are grieving the loss of the normal child they planned to have. This may be true, but the initial expression of such grieving may be to feel stuck on some part of the expected parenting experience that has been disrupted, not the entire package (figure 1). Asking a parent the simple question of what seems most challenging to them at the moment may yield clues to help them move forward. A parent may be worrying that the newly hired nanny speaks only Greek, and that you may advise sticking to one language for a while. A father may have viewed reading to his child as the essence of parenting, and may feel as though that pleasure will never happen, until he learns that one can read to a child who is deaf and gains confidence that he can do so. A mother may be fearful that she will be unable to learn auditory language stimulation techniques or sign language well enough to help her child (figure 2). The thought that the child will not hear music the usual way may feel paralyzing. Parents may feel panicked over the cost of hearing aids and therapy, and may not be able to hear more until they learn that funding may be available. They may worry that in-laws will attempt to lay etiological blame when they learn the diagnosis. Some may worry that any intervention such as hearing aids will interfere with religiously based healing. Finding out the specifics of how the loss of the planned child-rearing experience translates to the parent can provide a key to hand to the parents, to help them feel ready to move forward. In so doing, we learn about the family's home life, personal values, and beliefs about health and medical care. Sometimes we need to reveal a little

(THEY ARE DISTRAUGHT. THEY ARE MOURNING THE LOSS OF THE NORMAL BABY THEY THOUGHT THEY HAD.)
"YOUR BABY IS FORTUNATE THAT YOU ACTED ON THE SCREENING REFERRAL. HE DOES INDEED HAVE PARTIAL HEARING ON BOTH SIDES."
OH NO! SHE'LL PROBABLY TELL US WE SHOULD STICK TO ONE LANGUAGE, AND IT'S SO IMPORTANT TO MY WIFE THAT OUR SON LEARNS HER NATIVE GERMAN ALSO.
OH NO! I JUST WENT BACK TO WORK AND MY NEW BOSS WILL NEVER GIVE ME TIME OFF FOR ALL THE APPOINTMENTS MY BABY WILL NEED.

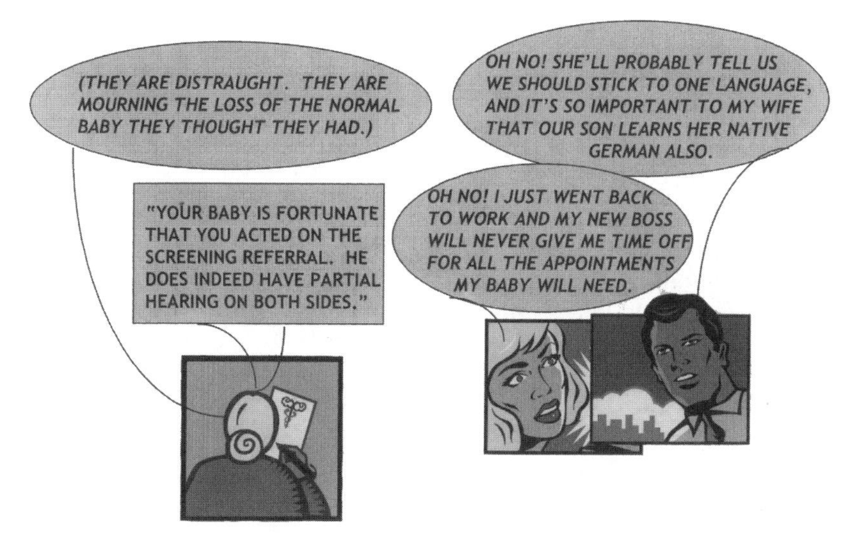

Figure 1. Audiologist's and parents' words and thoughts, as the diagnosis is imparted.

(I WISH I KNEW WHICH PART OF THE PROBLEM THEY ARE MOST WORRIED ABOUT.)
"YOUR BABY IS FORTUNATE THAT YOU ACTED ON THE SCREENING REFERRAL. HE DOES INDEED HAVE PARTIAL HEARING ON BOTH SIDES."
HOW WILL WE EVER BE ABLE TO AFFORD HEARING AIDS? PLUS I KNOW MY MOTHER WILL TRY TO PUT THE BLAME ON MY WIFE THAT THE BABY HAS A PROBLEM.
I'M SO AFRAID THAT I WON'T BE ABLE TO LEARN SIGN LANGUAGE FOR HIM.

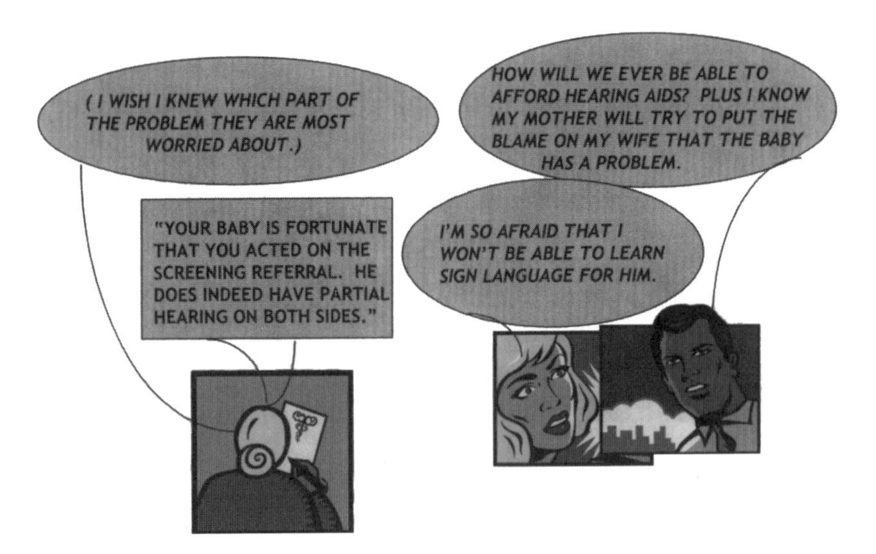

Figure 2. More words and thoughts from the audiologist and parents, as the diagnosis is imparted.

about ourselves in the process. If a family knows that we, as clinicians, place value and not judgment on the beliefs, worries, and experiences that people bring to new challenges, it will be easier for them to participate in a plan of care.

The top three most unhelpful things to say to parents who have just learned that their baby does not hear may be: "I know how you feel." (Doubtful! Even if you have been told something at least momentarily devastating about your own child in the past, these parents do not know that.); "It could be worse." (The baby will help them figure that out later, but not yet.); "You should be seen in Genetics to make sure this doesn't happen again." (WHAT? Such a comment conveys that their baby, this baby with whom they are hopelessly in love, has something so terrible that society will not value the child.).

Presenting inconclusive or partial test results to parents may put them in a special place of agony. As the comic strip philosopher Pogo once said, "The certainty of misery is better than the misery of uncertainty." Parents in this situation may feel helped by understanding what is clear from the test results so far, what is not yet known, how the missing information can be gained, and how much hope they can have. "Hope" takes many forms: hope that the next test will show normal hearing; hope that a medication, an operation, or hearing aids will restore normal hearing; or hope that their child will be healthy and intelligent. Providing reality-based hope may be the kindest and most helpful thing a clinician can do.

TESTING THE INFANT'S HEARING

A detailed manual for pediatric audiology test procedures is far beyond the scope of this presentation. A number of excellent books detail the procedures that a pediatric audiologist must have mastered in order to assess an infant's hearing status (for example, Hood 1998; Madell 1998; Hall 2000). A logical, if daunting, flow of test procedures following a referral from newborn hearing screening is presented in figure 3.

The Joint Committee on Infant Hearing (American Academy of Pediatrics 2000) position statement lists the following to be included in the test battery for infants under six months of age: history and parental report; frequency-specific electrophysiological measure of

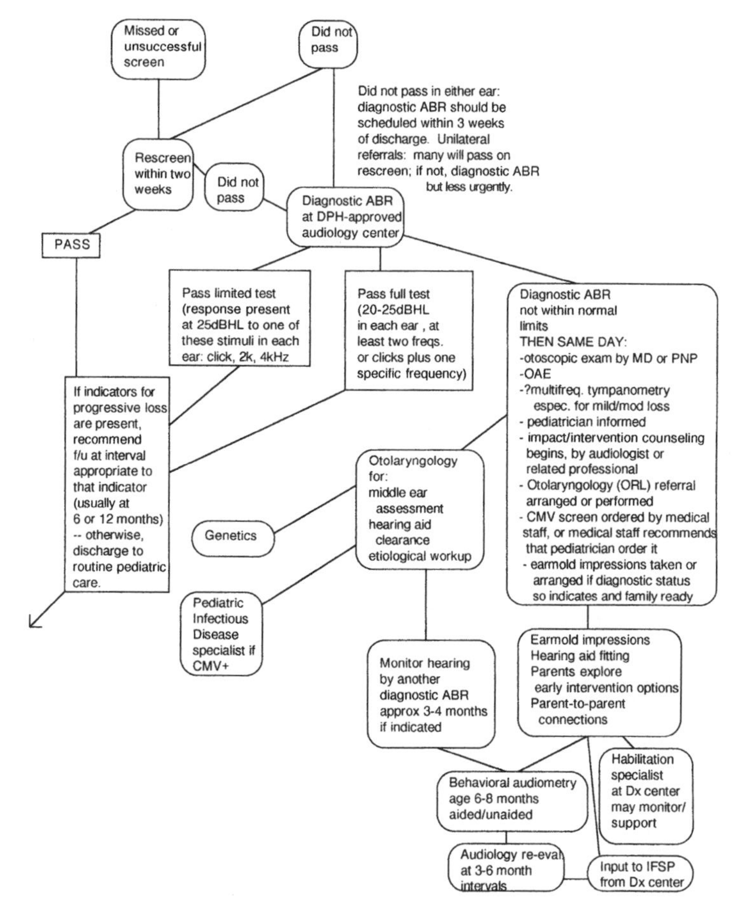

Figure 3. Detailed prospective follow-up for newborn hearing screening referrals.

thresholds; otoacoustic emissions; assessment of middle ear function using tympanometry with an appropriate probe frequency, reflectance, bone conduction ABR, and/or pneumatic otoscopy; acoustic reflex thresholds; and observation of behavioral responses to sounds. Rather than proceed down a list, however, the pediatric audiologist adopts a detective strategy most likely to yield a diagnosis in the most logical and efficient manner. The usual "first test" for a newborn referred from screening for a diagnostic audiological evaluation is the Auditory Brainstem Response (ABR) test, which must be frequency-specific unless it is conducted merely as a rescreen that turns out to be "passed." Ruling out ear canal occlusion or middle ear fluid before an unsedated sleep ABR, although a worthy goal, may be precluded by the starving and exhausted state in which the parents were instructed to bring the baby, in preparation to feed the baby and rock him to sleep for the test. If the ABR results do not confirm normal hearing, and/or if otoacoustic emissions are not normal, then assessment of outer and middle ear status on the day of the tests is essential.

Although an infant cannot give an accurate behavioral audiogram in the first weeks of life, parents of a baby even a few days old may be able to provide helpful impressions of the baby's behavioral responsiveness to sounds. Behavioral observation audiometry in an audiometric sound suite can and should help to corroborate or supplement physiological test results in a child with abnormal ABR findings. However, the chance of ruling out a mild hearing loss in an infant under six months of age by behavioral audiometric methods is poor, and so the first test session for infants up to six months of age usually is scheduled as an ABR, with OAE; tympanometry, and acoustic reflexes are needed the same day if the ABR results are not robustly normal. For babies several months old or older, when behavioral audiometric measures become more reliable, a typical setup of an audiometric sound suite for behavioral audiometry is shown in figure 4. When visual reinforcement audiometry (VRA) is used, the reinforcement can be kept to one side (ideally the side toward which the baby shows his first head-turn during the test, regardless of the side to which the sound was presented) or activated on either side. For either VRA or conditioned play audiometry, seating and positioning the child for optimal listening is essential. The child should be either comfortably on a lap but not sinking back into the parent's chest, or seated in his own chair with his feet firmly planted on a footrest rather than dangling and kicking in the air. If the child is in the parent's lap, the parent should wear an ear protection headset to dampen the test sounds so that the parent will not be giving clues to the baby to respond. If a child using conditioned play audiometry becomes uninterested before the test is over, adding the activation of a visual

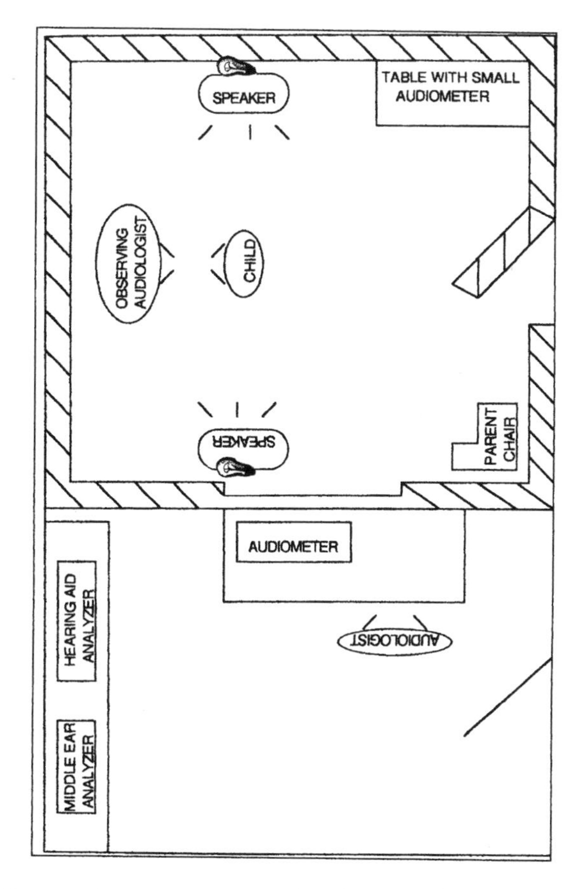

Figure 4. One working arrangement for visual reinforcement audiometry in a two-room audiometric sound suite.

reinforcer toy after each play audiometry response may help to revitalize the child's attention to the task long enough to finish the audiogram. Equipment can be arranged so that a single well-coordinated audiologist can perform the test in the same room with the child, activating both the stimulus and the visual reinforcer.

EFFECT OF ETIOLOGICAL FACTORS ON AUDIOLOGICAL PLAN

Knowledge about the specific etiologies of hearing loss in babies is mushrooming to the extent that the plan of audiological management may be shaped by knowing the likely cause of the hearing loss. The two causes of hearing loss in newborns that are becoming apparent, and that together account for a large portion of the 50% of deaf and hard of hearing babies with previously unknown etiologies, are connexin 26 mutations and asymptomatic congenital cytomegalovirus (CMV). Because most hearing losses associated with connexin 26 mutations are stable, whereas many associated with CMV are progressive, the frequency of retesting and the amount of reserve power prescribed in the hearing aids may both be influenced by the etiology.

Genetic advances and connexin 26. Advances in the understanding of the genetics of hearing loss are occurring so rapidly that one must check relevant journals and web sites frequently to learn of newly located or identified genes. Geneticists have been able to tell families with nonsyndromic deafness for some time when the pattern of inheritance of hearing loss in their particular family appears to be autosomal dominant. However, a guess at autosomal recessive inheritance, often without prior known family history of hearing loss, resulted primarily from process of elimination until recent location and identification of specific genes. The loci for over 60 genes for nonsyndromic sensorineural hearing loss have been found. Of these, 30 are autosomal dominant, 28 autosomal recessive, 5 X-linked, and 2 mitochondrial. Fifteen of the genes have been identified, ultimately leading to laboratory tests for mutations in these genes in specific human beings.

One particular gene has been unveiled as being responsible for approximately 50% of autosomal recessive nonsyndromic hearing loss, and a few cases of autosomal dominant hearing loss. The gene is GJB2 on chromosome 13, which encodes connexin 26, a gap junction protein which is plentiful in the cochlea. A change as small as the deletion of one guanine base from a string of six guanine molecules in a row on one little segment of the gene can cause hearing loss. Three percent of the general population carries one copy of a connexin 26 mutation (Korf 2000). There are several ways in which this gene can differ in individuals with hearing loss, when both copies (from the mother and father) of the gene are different from the typical pattern. A child with hearing loss might have inherited one copy of the mutated GJB2 gene from the mother and one copy from the father that is mutated in either the same way or a different way. When the mother and father each have one mutated copy, each of their children has a one in four chance of having hearing loss, if the pattern is one of true autosomal recessive inheritance. Kenna (2000) reported that of 57 children without an obvious cause for their hearing loss, 26 (46%) had connexin 26 mutations, 17 in both copies of the gene and 9 in one copy of the gene (these latter 9 children may have had no relationship between their connexin 26 status and their hearing loss, unless a single mutation can activate another process that causes hearing loss). The hearing loss varied from a mild high-frequency loss to a bilateral profound loss. Because deaf and hard of hearing children with the connexin 26 gene mutation typically do not have other physical anomalies, knowing about the genetic status early may help to eliminate the need for other diagnostic testing to get at the cause of the hearing loss or to look for other differences. Such advances in genetics make it incumbent on the audiologist to work ever more closely with the otolaryngologist and geneticist in the diagnostic process.

Congenital cytomegalovirus. A diagnostic stone only partially turned over at this point is that of cytomegalovirus (CMV) as a cause of hearing loss in infants. Newborns who are symptomatic for cytomegalovirus (CMV), based on such evidence as enlarged liver and spleen and elevated bilirubin, are tested for CMV early. These babies should be, and usually are, referred for serial audiological evaluations because of the high incidence of hearing loss which can be progressive. They may have other developmental challenges resulting from the CMV infection as well, and some are given a course of antiviral therapy in the first weeks of life to hold the virus at bay while neural substrates are developing (Nigro et al. 1994). However, significant numbers of newborns have congenital CMV infections which are not overtly symptomatic, yet can cause hearing loss which also can be progressive (Williamson et al. 1992). Figure 5 estimates the approximate numbers of children who may have hearing loss from congenital CMV, using population incidences of maternal infection, transmission

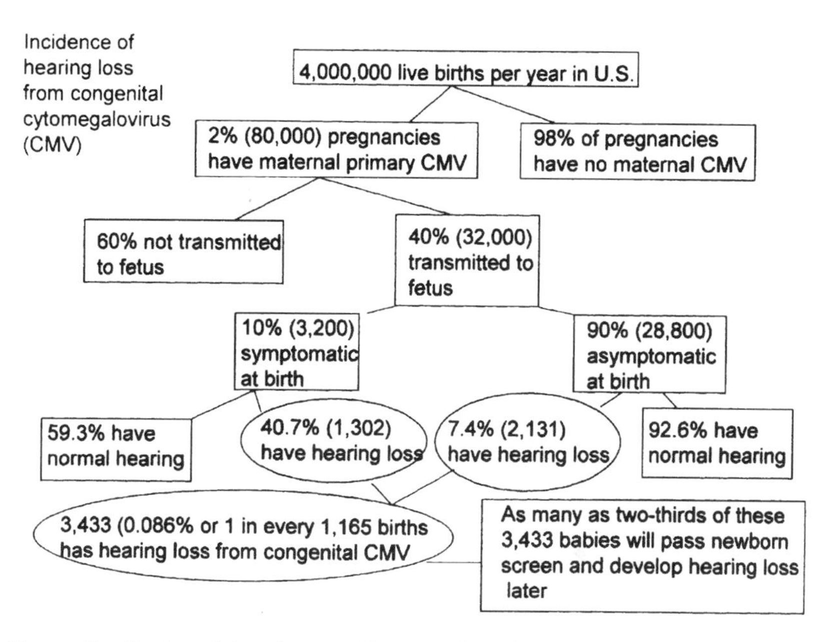

Figure 5. Projected incidence of hearing loss from congenital cytomegalovirus infections.

to the fetus, and presence of hearing loss as best estimates averaged over a variety of sources. By the time the hearing loss has been identified at several months of age or later in a child asymptomatic for CMV at birth, testing the child for evidence of past CMV infection does not succeed in ruling in CMV as the cause of the hearing loss, because the CMV infection could have been acquired postnatally in which case it would have been unrelated to the hearing loss.

It is clear that newborns with asymptomatic CMV infections should be referred for audiological monitoring even if they pass a newborn hearing screening test (Hicks et al. 1993). Figure 6 proposes a plan for audiological monitoring for infants with symptomatic vs. asymptomatic congenital CMV. However, the newborns with asymptomatic CMV are not identified because universal newborn screening for CMV is not included in the usual menu of newborn blood screening tests, and in fact the screening test for CMV is costlier than a newborn hearing screening test. Accordingly, at the present time, asymptomatic congenital CMV remains a likely reason for many of the deaf and hard of hearing children from the 50% of "unknown etiologies," after children with connexin 26 mutation are identified from that mix.

When a baby's hearing loss has an etiology that predisposes it to have a progressive hearing loss, the audiologist's responsibilities to that child and family are increased. Among these responsibilities are

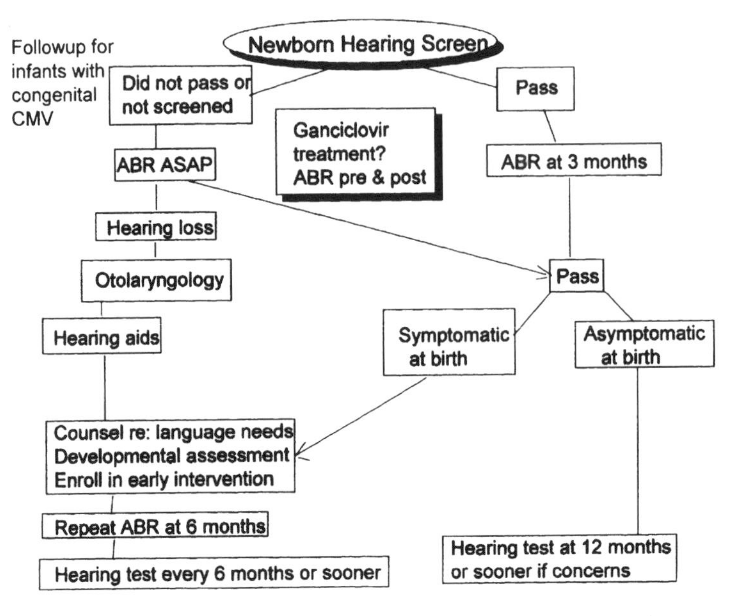

Figure 6. Recommended audiological monitoring for infants with congenital cytomegalovirus infections.

providing accurate frequency-specific tests on a timely schedule, monitoring middle ear status, coordinating audiology appointments with otolaryngology visits, recommending hearing aids with reserve power and adjusting them carefully, informing the family of resources available in case hearing worsens, and watching out for the child's emotional well-being and educational needs.

Auditory dys-synchrony. A further development that has complicated, yet elucidated, the diagnostic scene for newborns is the recently evolving science of identifying cases of auditory dys-synchrony ("auditory neuropathy," Starr et al. 1996). Children with this condition have evidence of hair cell activity in the cochlea, but do not have organized discharge of auditory neurons as a result of that cochlear activity. The evidence for cochlear activity in these children comes reliably from the presence of a prolonged cochlear microphonic response in their auditory brainstem response (ABR) tracings, followed by a lack of ABR waves. The cochlear microphonic is distinguished from stimulus artifact by running a control tracing with the insert phone tubing pinched, which makes the cochlear microphonic disappear from the tracing. The cochlear microphonic is distinguishable from auditory neural responses because neural evoked potentials do not reverse polarity when one reverses the polarity of the click stimulus from rarefaction to condensation, whereas the cochlear microphonic response does reverse polarity with reversals in stimulus polarity. This reversal can be seen in Figure 7, recorded from a nine-month old girl in our clinic with auditory dys-synchrony.

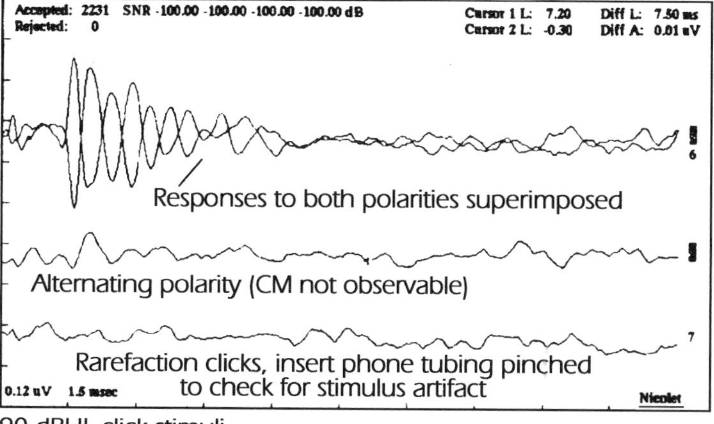

Figure 7. Auditory Brainstem Response tracings from a nine-month old child with auditory dys-synchrony ("auditory neuropathy").

Children with auditory dys-synchrony present a confusing pattern of auditory behaviors and auditory test results. They have a cochlear microphonic response, but no true ABR waveforms. They often have otoacoustic emissions, providing further evidence of cochlear activity, although they may lose their otoacoustic emissions over the first few months of life while retaining the cochlear microphonic. To date it appears that in general they do not have acoustic (stapedial) reflexes. Hearing aids do not provide the benefit expected from their pure tone audiogram. In our growing clinic population of over 30 children with auditory dys-synchrony, most have the findings bilaterally but a few unilaterally.

Although a few children with this condition may have true neuropathy, many are thought to have missing or ineffective inner hair cells or synaptic insufficiency in the generation of the compound action potential of the auditory nerve. Evidence that the auditory nerve itself has the potential to be functional comes partly from the growing numbers of children with auditory dys-synchrony who hear well with cochlear implants (Shallop et al. 2001).

Two aspects of auditory dys-synchrony render it the most difficult of the various diagnoses of hearing loss for parents to understand and accept. First, the audiologist is unable to give them a prognosis for future development of the functional use of hearing. Some children with auditory dys-synchrony improve in their auditory responsiveness to the point that they can develop useful spoken language. Others remain functionally deaf, and need to rely on visual language not only as a jump-start but as a continuing means of language input. Second, parents are confused by the pattern of auditory behaviors typical of auditory dys-synchrony. Children with this condition who have relatively good pure tone audiograms still do not understand speech clearly, particularly in noise. Children with this condition who have severe or profound loss on their audiograms still show occasional, unpredictable responses to sounds in the environment that they should not be able to hear based on their audiogram, and may have what parents call "good hearing days" and "bad hearing days." These mismatches between the audiogram and the auditory behavior confound the audiologist, the otolaryngologist, and the parent. At all times, the parents' observations of the child's responses to sounds should be queried and respected in these children.

Our experience has taught us that children with auditory dys-synchrony are presenting to our audiology service in three different ways. The first and largest group consists of infants referred by newborn ABR screen who would not otherwise have been suspected of having an auditory disorder at birth. Their ABRs show only cochlear microphonics without further ABR waves. Tympanograms with

1000Hz probe tones are recorded to rule out middle ear fluid, and acoustic reflexes (absent) and otoacoustic emissions (present or absent) are recorded. An inventory of parental observations of responses to sounds is gathered. A second group consists of "passed" newborns whose hearing screen in the hospital was accomplished using otoacoustic emissions, yet the parent suspects hearing loss and brings the baby in. The test battery is the same as for the first group. A third, much smaller, group presenting to our clinic has been children age three to five years with partial hearing loss who are not progressing well in acquiring spoken language using hearing aids in oral preschool programs, and turn out to have previously undiagnosed auditory dys-synchrony.

The management of children with auditory dys-synchrony includes careful explanation to the parents of what is known and what is not known about the future of their child's hearing, what will be done to delineate the development of hearing abilities, and encouragement to introduce a visual language system to the child while fostering any auditory responsiveness that develops. Cochlear implantation can be considered at age two years or later if functional hearing has not shown strong signs of developing. At some point soon, electrophysiological measures may emerge that help predict which children with auditory dys-synchrony will "recover" and which should remain with visual language systems or proceed to the option of a cochlear implant.

We must recall that when we set out to test hearing in all newborns, we realized that we would learn a great deal about newborn hearing, and auditory dys-synchrony is one of the phenomena we are learning about. We also have learned why, ten and twenty years ago, parents swore their child used to hear better or worse than at the time of diagnosis, and why parents swore that their child occasionally responded to sounds that their audiogram would not allow them to hear. The parents were right, although we explained away their anecdotes saying it was denial, response to vibrations or subtle visual cues, or wishful thinking. Parents, after all, are the best audiologists.

REFERENCES

American Academy of Pediatrics. 1992. The medical home (RE9262, policy statement), *Pediatrics* 90(5):774.

American Academy of Pediatrics. 2000. Principles and guidelines for early hearing detection and intervention programs (Joint Committee on Infant Hearing - Year 2000 position statement). http://www.aap.org/policy/jcihyr2000.pdf.

Hall, J. W. III. 2000. *Handbook of Otoacoustic Emissions.* San Diego: Singular.

Hicks, T., Fowler, K., Richardson, M., Dahle, A., Adams, L., and Pass, R. 1993. Congenital cytomegalovirus infection and neonatal auditory screening. *The Journal of Pediatrics* 123(5):779–82.

Hood, L. J. 1998. *Clinical Applications of the Auditory Brainstem Response.* Delmar Publishers.

Kenna, M. A. 2000. Incidence of connexin 26 mutations in children with non-syndromic hearing loss. Personal communication.

Korf, B. R. 2000. *Human Genetics: A Problem-Based Approach.* 2nd edition. London: Blackwell Science.

Madell, J. R. 1998. *Behavioral Evaluation of Hearing in Infants and Young Children.* New York: Thieme.

Nigro, G., Scholz, H., and Bartmann, U. 1994. Ganciclovir therapy for symptomatic congenital cytomegalovirus infection in infants: A two-regimen experience. *Journal of Pediatrics* 124(2):318–22.

Shallop, J., Fabry, L., Colin, D., Peterson, A., and Stoeckel, R. 2001. Cochlear implants in patients with auditory neuropathy. Presented at Cochlear Implants in Children, 8th Symposium, Los Angeles.

Starr, A., Picton, T. W., Sininger, Y., Hood, L. J., and Berlin, C. I. 1996. Auditory neuropathy. *Brain* 119:741–53.

Williamson, W. D., Demmler, G. J., Percy, A. K., and Catlin, F. I. 1992. Progressive hearing loss in infants with asymptomatic congenital cytomegalovirus infection. *Pediatrics* 90(6):862–66.

Chapter ▪ 4

Staying Family-Centered

Jackson Roush

For most families, the journey into deafness begins with the diagnosis of permanent hearing loss. Many families vividly recall the circumstances surrounding this event. The phrases "sensorineural hearing loss," "no medical treatment," "need for hearing aids and special services" are often indelible. Much has been said and written about the dynamics of this encounter (Luterman 1979; 1984). Unfortunately, parent surveys and testimonials often point to a mismatch between parent perceptions and those of professionals (Martin et al. 1987). One of the few studies to examine the diagnostic encounter using qualitative research methods was a master's thesis conducted at Emerson College under the direction of David Luterman. Soon after the initial diagnosis, Lerner (1988) interviewed family members and professionals to examine what parents "heard" in comparison to what the audiologist thought he or she had communicated. The following is a brief quotation from the mother of a newly identified infant:

> I think we left that day with no reason to be hopeful. There was a lot [the audiologist] could have told us or given us. He could have said to us that "deaf isn't what deaf used to be, because with hearing aids being what they are, kids can do a lot with their residual hearing." He really didn't give us any reason to be hopeful.

I read this transcript with genuine interest because the audiologist, in this case, happened to be me. This was several years ago, but I was not a new graduate and I was not inexperienced at working with families. In fact, I considered myself skilled at communicating with families. Although I reacted defensively at first, the experience marked the beginning of a longstanding interest in parent-professional communication and how we, as professionals, can improve our competency in this area.

For the past ten years, in collaboration with colleagues and students at the University of North Carolina at Chapel Hill, we have undertaken several projects aimed at exploring various aspects of "family-centered early intervention" and what that means to professionals and to family members. We have also learned a great deal from the work of others. This chapter will examine some of the relevant literature and will conclude with an examination of the specific contexts encountered clinically by audiologists and early intervention personnel during the weeks and months from screening to intervention.

HISTORICAL AND LEGISLATIVE PERSPECTIVES

For many years, traditional early intervention was a child-focused endeavor, with a primary purpose of enhancing developmental outcomes for young children with disabilities. According to Trivette and colleagues (Trivette et al. 1995), the term "family centered" was first used in the health care field in the 1960s in an effort to improve obstetric and nursing practices. Bronfenbrenner (1975) is credited with applying the term to early intervention in the 1970s to increase the level of parent participation in early education.

Beginning in the 1980s, contemporary views of "best practice" resulted in federal and state legislation aimed at promoting family-centered practices. For the first time, a multidisciplinary team evaluation resulting in an Individualized Family Service Plan (IFSP) is required, in addition to information about the child, documentation of a family's strengths and needs, services to be provided to the family, and specification of intended outcomes. Beginning with Public Law 99-457 in 1986, family-centered services were no longer optional but required by law.

As federal and state mandates began to influence practices nationwide, Don Bailey and colleagues at the Frank Porter Graham Child Development Center at the University of North Carolina and Carl Dunst and colleagues at the Western Carolina Center were among the first to examine the shift toward family-centered services. Not surprisingly, they found considerable variability in how family-centered practices were defined and implemented (Bailey et al. 1992; Dunst et al. 1991; Mahoney, O'Sullivan, and Dennebaum 1990). To facilitate comparison of practice patterns, Dunst et al. (1991) described four models for working with families: professionally centered, family-allied, family-focused, and family-centered. According to Dunst and colleagues, proponents of professionally centered models view professionals as experts who determine child and family needs from their own, as opposed to a family's, perspective. In family-allied models, families are seen as agents of professionals and are enlisted to implement interventions that professionals deem important and necessary for optimal child and family functioning. Advocates of family-focused models view families as consumers of professional services and assist families in choosing among options that professionals consider necessary for best meeting child and family needs. In contrast, proponents of family-centered models view professionals as instruments of families and intervene in ways that are individualized, flexible, and responsive, and in ways that support and strengthen family functioning. In advocating for this latter approach, Dunst and colleagues (Dunst et al. 1991; Trivette et al. 1995) have argued for major changes in how service delivery systems are organized and operated, and in how practitioners view their roles and responsibilities in working with children and families. Likewise, Bailey et al. (1998) have urged the use of family outcomes (in addition to child outcomes) for determining the extent to which family-centered practices are implemented. In order to assess family outcomes, Bailey and colleagues have developed a framework around which program evaluation and efficacy research can be conducted. More recently, Dunst (2000) has proposed an expanded service delivery model focusing on the social systems and environmental variables associated with "development enhancing and family-strengthening consequences." This model includes children's learning opportunities, supports for parenting, and family/community supports provided within a family-centered framework.

The ensuing years have witnessed several re-authorizations of the federal mandate for family-centered early intervention that are now contained in Part C of the Individuals with Disabilities Education Act (IDEA). The most fundamental principle of this legislation is a focus on parental decision-making and individualized choices for families throughout the delivery of early intervention services.

EVALUATING FAMILY-CENTERED PRACTICES

Although it is evident from the literature that professionals value a family-centered approach, there appears to be substantial disparity between actual and ideal practices (Bailey et al. 1992; Crais and Wilson 1996; Dunst, et al. 1991; Mahoney et al. 1990). Facilitating a family-centered approach requires careful examination of parent-professional communication and the dynamics of each context that brings parents and professionals together. Simeonsson and colleagues (1996) suggest that early intervention services may be viewed as an intervention cycle composed of discrete elements including referral, assessment, intervention planning, service implementation, and follow up.

Each element involves a succession of "encounters" that children and families have with professionals, and each encounter is defined by mutual expectations, roles, and activities for both families and service providers. Our encounters with deaf and hard-of-hearing children and their families include each component of this intervention cycle. Initially they revolve around the screening and diagnostic process and later with the selection and fitting of sensory devices and delivery of early intervention services. Along the way, professionals impart information and offer choices to families. For the audiologist, the parent-professional relationship often begins with a diagnostic assessment, in many cases on referral from a newborn hearing-screening program. Regrettably, we continue to hear testimonials from some parents regarding experiences with audiologists who were perceived as indifferent or insensitive to their needs early on, or in other cases (as in my own experience noted above) were well-intentioned but missed the mark on what the family needed at the time. On the other hand, when supportive and mutually satisfying relationships occur, the audiologist is considered by many families to be a supportive and trusted collaborator (Roush 2000).

The advantages of a collaborative approach between parents and professionals are especially evident during the process of evaluating benefits of hearing aids and other sensory devices. Although specific procedures have been developed for the selection of hearing aid electroacoustic characteristics (Seewald et al 1997), careful observation of the child is still needed (Harrison 2000). Parents not only know the child better than anyone else, their observations occur in natural environments. Consequently, their input can help evaluate current performance and guide the decision-making process regarding future interventions. Systematic observation by parents and caretakers is especially critical when decisions need to be made regarding if and when to move a young child from acoustic amplification to cochlear implantation. On a more basic level, parents and caregivers ultimately determine how well the instruments function and, indeed, whether they are used at all. Even with the most competent clinical management, audiologic intervention efforts cannot be optimized without strong parent-professional collaboration.

Despite anecdotal reports and survey literature on the perceived benefits of parent-professional collaboration, little is known about the extent to which parents and professionals actually employ family-centered practices, and if they do, which practices are preferred by families and professionals. Recently, Crais and Belardi (1999) reviewed the early intervention literature on parent participation in the assessment process. Although not limited specifically to children with hearing loss, their findings are clearly relevant. Three conclusions emerged.

First, it was shown that parents have historically served primarily as informants and observers in assessment, having veto power over decisions made by professionals about intervention goals, but often deferring to professionals with little input to decision making. A second conclusion across several studies was that despite limited opportunities for parental decision-making in the assessment process, parents have been generally satisfied with the roles available to them. But as the authors also note, families may have been under-informed consumers during the delivery of early intervention services because they simply have not been aware of alternative practices (Porter et al. 1995). The third, and perhaps most significant conclusion, was that both families and professionals have perceived a gap between actual and ideal practices. Crais and Belardi also surveyed parents and early intervention personnel to explore family and professional perceptions regarding current and ideal ways families participate in child assessment. The survey data are encouraging in that a number of the family-centered principles advocated in the literature were, in fact, being used by the professionals they surveyed. There was also evidence of congruence between families and professionals on a number of preferred practices. Their findings revealed, however, that gaps between actual and ideal practices continue to persist in several key areas. For example from both parents' and professionals' perspectives, more time should be devoted to identifying the specific steps in the planning process, encouraging a more active role for parents in interpreting their child's behaviors, and determining when and where assessment results are discussed.

PROFESSIONAL PERSPECTIVES ON FAMILY-CENTERED PRACTICES

The work of Crais and Belardi (1999) provides a useful vantage point from which to consider services to newly identified infants and toddlers with hearing loss and their families. Do we view parents primarily as informants or do we provide them with the information they need to make their own decisions? Some findings from a nationwide survey may suggest the former. Roush, Harrison, and Palsha (1991) investigated attitudes and opinions of early intervention professionals regarding parent collaboration in the planning and implementation of goals and services for deaf and hard-of-hearing infants and toddlers and their families. The results of the study suggest that practitioners working with young deaf and hard-of-hearing children place a high value on the need for and desirability of family-centered intervention. But the study also revealed that when a discrepancy exists between parent and professional priorities, many professionals are reluctant to defer to family preferences.

Educational Preparation of Audiologists and Early Intervention Specialists

Professional attitudes are undoubtedly shaped by experiences at the pre-service level. In order to learn more about the status of course work and practicum related to early intervention and working with families, Roush et al. (1992) conducted a nationwide survey of college and university programs in education of the deaf. Curriculum content and practicum experiences with infants and toddlers and their families were examined as well as general comments and recommendations of program directors. In general, program directors indicated that they value family-centered early intervention, but they also noted substantial difficulties in the expansion of pre-service curricula focusing on early intervention and working with families. Educators report that program requirements are already extensive, and that other topic areas are competing for further attention. In addition, certification constraints in some states complicate the development of infant-toddler and preschool specializations within traditional deaf education programs.

Similar findings have been noted in studies that have looked at educational preparation of audiologists. In a nationwide survey of graduate education for audiologists, Oyler and Matkin (1987) surveyed program directors and recently certified audiologists, asking them to evaluate their educational experiences in pediatric audiology. In the component of the study that dealt with parent-professional relations, it was interesting to note that three-fourths of the respondents indicated their graduate programs offered no course work dealing specifically with counseling parents and family members. Among newly certified audiologists, fewer than one in four had taken a course related to working with families. Not surprisingly, most expressed feeling ill-prepared to work with young children and their families.

These results are consistent with those of McCarthy and colleagues (1986) who surveyed program directors in communication disorders departments and found substantial variability in course offerings, course content, and program requirements. The majority, nearly three-fourths, believed that a course in counseling should be offered by the communicative disorders department and should be required at the graduate level. But few programs (12%) offered such courses and practicum within their academic units. As the authors point out, courses from other departments are better than none at all, but they are unlikely to include information specific to counseling families with deaf and hard-of-hearing children.

More recent surveys indicate little evidence of change. The results of Culpepper, Mendel, and McCarthy's (1994) 10-year follow-up study to the original McCarthy et al. (1986) survey were remarkably similar. An even more recent survey by Crandell (1997) indicated that only 18% of the students graduating from an audiology program had course work in counseling. It is little surprise that fewer than half of the audiologists surveyed by Martin, Bar, and Bernstein (1992) considered themselves well-prepared in the area of counseling. Perhaps as the audiology curriculum expands in the process of moving toward doctoral entry level, improvements will be seen. There is encouraging preliminary evidence from a study by English, Mendel, and Rojeski, (1999) indicating that Au.D. students showed positive changes in their counseling skills as a result of specialized course work.

ADVICE FROM FAMILIES

When asked, families are willing to share their experiences regarding parent-professional practices and how they can be improved. For example, Roush (2000) reported a survey of families who were receiving a free first-year membership in the Alexander Graham Bell Association. The children were recently identified and, because of the free membership, the families were probably more diverse than the A.G. Bell membership at large. This was not, however, a random sample and in that sense, not based on a scientific survey method. Still, their comments were interesting and thought-provoking. Ninety-seven families responded to a questionnaire designed to solicit opinions regarding initial intervention and audiology services. Early intervention services were defined as professional services provided by special educators, speech-language pathologists, teachers of the hearing impaired, or other professionals providing services related to education or communication. Parents were asked to respond separately to the same questions related to both early intervention and audiology service providers. Audiology services included assessment, as well as hearing aid related services, and the manner in which those services were rendered. Specifically parents were asked to respond to several questions regarding what was most and least helpful to them in the early stages of assessment and intervention. Of particular interest were responses to the following question: "What is the single most important thing for audiologists to consider when planning services for families with newly identified deaf and hard-of-hearing children?" The same question was asked with reference to early intervention specialists. For both professional disciplines, the advice from parents was similar: In the early stages parents want objective information regarding all options so they can make well informed decisions; they want professionals to be sensitive to the emotional shock and upheaval they are experiencing; and they want professionals to be honest and realistic, but hopeful, in their prognosis. Many also expressed a need for greater availability of specialized intervention services and more contact with other parents. Interestingly, these are the same themes echoed in other studies (e.g. Luterman 1986; Luterman and Kurtzer-White 1999; Roush and Matkin 1994).

What About Dissatisfied Families?

Although most families appear to want a collaborative relationship with professionals, some parents will challenge even the most family-centered clinicians. Experienced practitioners have all encountered families whose requests (or in some cases "demands") are regarded as inappropriate or unreasonable. Eventually we must question how far professionals should be expected to go in yielding to parental wishes. Certainly, professionals must be committed to providing the highest level of care, according to existing standards of "best practice." Inevitably though, parent preferences regarding hearing aid selection, intervention options, or other considerations will, at times, create parent-professional conflict. Fortunately, these dilemmas are often temporary, especially if clinicians pay close attention to factors that may underlie the family's point of view. Luterman (1985) encourages professionals to "listen for affect" when responding to parents' questions and comments. The issue of pursuing a smaller hearing aid, for example, may actually reflect the family's difficulty accepting the appearance of the instrument. In such a case, the audiologist would be wise to attend to those needs rather than responding only to the technical issues of acoustic feedback and output limitation. In addition, a parent support group can often facilitate the process of constructive acceptance. Unfortunately, there is not a program like Emerson's Thayer-Lindsley Nursery available to every parent! But professionals in any city can maintain a list of parents willing to provide peer support to families of newly identified children. This approach may be especially constructive when there is an apparent mismatch between parent and professional perspectives.

INFORMING AND SUPPORTING FAMILIES

There are several recurring scenarios during the early stages of identification, assessment, and intervention. Although each family is unique, most face similar circumstances. First, families must be informed of screening results and eventually of diagnostic findings. Those with a child found to have permanent hearing loss face decisions regarding the use of hearing aids and other sensory devices. Decisions will also be needed regarding options for early intervention. These are emotionally demanding times for families and they challenge the counseling skills of even the most seasoned clinicians. Since families and clinicians are all different there is no simple formula for how best to approach each scenario. But there are fundamental issues underlying each set of circumstances that transcend individual differences among families and professionals.

Reporting Results of Screening and Arranging for Follow Up

Universal newborn hearing screening is expanding rapidly throughout the nation. As a result, thousands of babies are screened every day and thousands of parents receive the news of a screening outcome. Most programs inform parents of screening results prior to hospital discharge, but some choose to wait a few days in order to allow families time to recover from the delivery and enjoy the initial bonding period without the anxiety of a possible hearing loss. Unfortunately, any delay increases the chances of babies being lost to follow up, especially in urban areas or when there are linguistic or cultural barriers. Clearly, there are important advantages to informing families during the birth admission, but care must be taken in how the information is delivered. Fortunately, most infants referred for retesting will turn out to have normal hearing. This fact needs to be clearly communicated to parents when initial screening results are reported, but reassurance must be balanced with sufficient emphasis on the importance of returning for follow up. Still, many programs prefer to avoid the terms "fail" or "failure" when reporting a screening outcome, opting instead for terminology such as "did not pass," or simply "refer." Others believe that a "failed screening" is more likely to encourage follow up.

Programs also vary with regard to who delivers the information. In many programs this responsibility is assigned to a nurse; however, some opt to have an audiologist deliver the information when screening results are abnormal. Regardless of who is assigned this responsibility, that person must fully appreciate the impact of this news. Anecdotal reports indicate that communication with families is, at times, handled with indifference or lack of information. For every program, the decisions of who informs families and how they convey this information are of utmost importance. If the designated individual is not an audiologist, he or she must be well-informed about audiologic assessment, intervention options, and issues that may be raised by the family. In-service education of nursing staff or other screening personnel is essential to insure that family members are provided with accurate information delivered in a manner that is considerate of their emotional needs. Parents should also be provided with access to further information in case they have questions prior to their return visit (Roush in press).

The issue of how and when screening results are reported also has implications for families whose children turn out to have normal hearing. This is another area where Luterman and colleagues have advised caution (Luterman and Kurtzer-White 1999). Fortunately, pass rates with automated ABR in many programs are now approaching 99% and consequently, the number of families unnecessarily inconvenienced or upset is declining. In addition, a recent study indicated that over 90% of the mothers in a well-baby nursery felt positive about universal newborn hearing screening (Clemens, Davis, and Bailey 2000). Similar findings have been reported elsewhere in the United States (Uzcategui and Yoshinaga-Itano 1997) and in the United Kingdom (Watkin et al. 1998). Still, group data are of little relevance to a given family. As Finitzo has said, "we get it right or wrong, one family at a time" (Hayes, et al. 1999). Childbirth is a momentous occasion for families. Screening personnel must never lose sight of their potential impact on this important event.

Informing Families of Diagnostic Results

Our ever-expanding technological capabilities combined with the growth of universal infant hearing screening have resulted in fundamental changes in how and when the diagnosis occurs. In contrast to earlier times when the audiologic assessment confirmed parental suspicions, the news now comes as a surprise to most families. Test results that may be unequivocal to professionals based on objective physiologic measures are, in the absence of direct evidence, difficult for parents to comprehend and accept. Clinicians must be prepared to respond to a broad range of questions including some that would appear irrelevant to the immediate circumstances. Recently, the only question asked by the mother of a three-week-old infant at our university hospital on the day of diagnosis was: "How will other children react to her hearing aids when she's a teenager?" Clearly there is no counseling template that can be applied at the time of diagnosis.

In an effort to focus on what parents need to know as opposed to what we want to tell them, Luterman has emphasized the importance of meeting parents where they are at each point. In addition to delivering information clearly and accurately with sensitivity to the impact of this news, it is important to remember that the child's degree of hearing loss is unrelated to the parents' level of emotional upheaval. For some families, the diagnosis of a mild or even unilateral hearing loss may be emotionally traumatic. Parents typically have many questions regarding the nature of their child's hearing loss and how they should proceed with intervention (Martin, Krall, and O'Neill 1989). For all families it is crucial that they leave the diagnostic evaluation with hope, based on the knowledge that much can and will be done for their child. Referral to a parent support group or to individual parents willing to provide peer support can be especially valuable at this time (Luterman and Kurtzer-White 1999).

DECISIONS REGARDING HEARING AID SELECTION/FITTING

Once the necessary medical and audiologic assessments have been completed, it is possible to proceed with hearing aid selection and fitting. The Joint Committee on Infant Hearing Year 2000 Position Statement (JCIH 2000) recommends that infants with no medical contraindications begin use of amplification within one month after confirmation of the hearing loss. But will all families be ready to move ahead that soon? For nearly all parents, this is a stressful and uncertain period with profound implications for the entire family. Some families will be ready to proceed immediately while others will need additional time. When parents were asked to indicate the optimal time interval from diagnosis to hearing aid fitting, Sjoblad (1997) found that nearly three-fourths of the parents surveyed said 3 to 4 weeks, but approximately one-fourth believed that 1 to 3 months was optimal. This finding underscores the natural variability among families and the importance of not assuming that all will want to proceed at the same pace. It may also, however, reflect the need for better counseling and/or peer support. That is, families who favored a longer delay may have lacked the information they needed to proceed comfortably with intervention.

An issue rarely discussed but clearly on the minds of most parents is the issue of appearance (recall from the earlier anecdote that this was the first issue on the mind of one parent on the day of diagnosis). Sjoblad (1997) reported that over half of the parent respondents expressed concern about the appearance of the devices. Nearly two-thirds also expressed concerns about the perceived benefits of amplification. Fortunately, for over half the respondents, perceptions regarding both appearance and benefit were more positive over time and only a small fraction (less than 5%) felt less positive over time.

Minimizing Delays from Diagnosis to Intervention

Although some delays are inevitable and for some families may be preferred, surveys have revealed a tremendous range in the time interval from diagnosis to intervention. In an effort to better understand the reasons for these delays, Harrison and Roush (1996) asked parents the following question: "If there was a delay of twelve weeks or more between diagnosis of the hearing loss and fitting of hearing aids or initiation of intervention services, what were the reasons?" The most frequently cited reasons were: (1) delays due to third-party payment or eligibility reviews; (2) delays due to the child's illness, including otitis media; (3) delays due to recommendations for further audiologic assessment; and (4) delays in achieving an appropriate hearing aid fitting. In a follow-up study, Sjoblad (1997) found a median delay of only two months from diagnosis to hearing aid fitting, but the range was over eight months. Reasons for delay were again probed, this time if there was a delay of more than one month. The reasons most frequently cited included: need for further audiologic assessment; problems with availability of return appointments; illness of the child; and problems with hearing aid fitting or earmolds. Although these problems are not easily solved, it is encouraging that many are potentially within our control. In particular, clinicians who agree to serve the infant population must have the necessary instrumentation as well as the knowledge and skills required to provide comprehensive diagnostic and audiologic intervention. This includes frequency-specific ABR and probe tube microphone measurements in conjunction with a fitting strategy appropriate for young children (see Seewald, Chapter 5, this text). Timely return visits must be ensured with reasonable effort to provide appointment times that allow multiple family members to be present at follow-up visits.

DECISIONS REGARDING EARLY INTERVENTION

Maximizing developmental language outcomes for young children with hearing loss requires that intervention begin soon after the hearing loss has been identified (Yoshinaga-Itano et al. 1998; Carney and Moeller 1998). But in order to make informed decisions regarding intervention, families need information that is objective, culturally sensitive, and considerate of their emotional state (Luterman 1985; Luterman and Kurtzer-White 1999). Thus, audiologists who work with infants must be familiar with legislative mandates as well as state and local referral procedures. Moreover, they must provide unbiased information regarding intervention options. The most important issue is not necessarily the initial decisions made by families but how freely they can revise the plan as they acquire more information and greater confidence. This entails a philosophical orientation that encourages families to make their own decisions and for professionals to support them in this process.

CONCLUSIONS

Professionals working with young deaf and hard-of-hearing children and their families are faced with many opportunities to be, or not to be, family centered. Putting family priorities first requires a reexamination of traditional practices and a willingness to step out of traditional roles. Of course, there are many situations that require the audiologist to be "in charge," particularly those concerning the selection and application of diagnostic procedures and other technical matters. But along the way, we must listen carefully to what families are telling us, with a readiness to perform our clinical roles in a manner, and at a pace, consistent with their priorities. For over 40 years, Luterman has encouraged us to explore the value of looking beyond the surface level in our work with families. Achieving a successful balance between "content" and "affect," between the technological and interpersonal demands of our work, is our single greatest professional challenge. Within that challenge, however, is the key to healthy parent-professional relationships and positive long-term outcomes for children, families, and professionals.

REFERENCES

Bailey, D. B., Buysee, V., Edmundson, R., and Smith, T. M. 1992. Creating family- centered services in early intervention: Perceptions of professionals in four states. *Exceptional Children* 58:298–309.

Bailey, D. B., McWilliam, R., Aytch Darkes, L., Hebbeler, K., Simeonsson, R., Spiker, D., and Wagner, M. 1998. Family outcomes in early intervention: A framework for program evaluation and efficacy research. *Exceptional Children* 64:313–28.

Boyd, K., Dunst, C. J., Hamby, D. W., and Trivette, C. M. 1996. Family oriented program models, helpgiving practices, and parental control appraisals. *Exceptional Children* __:237–48.

Carney, A., and Moeller, M. P. 1998. Treatment efficacy: Hearing loss in children. *Journal of Speech and Hearing Research* 41:S61–84.

Clemens, C. J., Davis, S. A., and Bailey, A. R. 2000. The false-positive in universal newborn hearing screening. *Pediatrics* 106(1):E7.

Crais, E., and Belardi, C. 1999. Family participation in child assessment: Perceptions of families and professionals. *Infant-Toddler Intervention* 6:209–38.

Crais, E., and Wilson, L. 1996. The role of parents in child assessment: Self-evaluation by practicing professionals. *Infant-Toddler Intervention* 9:209–38.

Crandell, C. 1997. An update on counseling instruction within audiology training programs. *Journal of the Academy of Rehabilitative Audiology* 30:1–10.

Culpepper, B., Mendel, L., and McCarthy, P. 1994. Counseling experience and training offered by ESB accredited programs. *Asha* 36:55–64.

Dunst, C. J. 2000. Revisiting "Rethinking early intervention." *Topics in Early Childhood Special Education* 20:95–104.

Dunst, C. J., Johanson, C., Trivette, C. M., and Hamby, D. 1991. Family-oriented early intervention policies and practices: Family-centered or not? *Exceptional Children* 58:115–26.

Harrison, M. 2000. How do we know we've got it right?: Observing performance with amplification. In *A Sound Foundation Through Early Amplification*, eds. R. Seewald, and A. G. Phonak.

Harrison, M., and Roush, J. 1996. Age of suspicion, identification and intervention for infants and young children with hearing loss: A national study. *Ear and Hearing* 17:55–62.
Joint Committee on Infant Hearing Year 2000 Position Statement 2000. *Audiology Today* August, Special Issue:6–27.
Luterman, D. 1979. *Counseling Parents of Hearing Impaired Children.* Boston: Little Brown.
Luterman, D. 1985. The denial mechanism. *Ear and Hearing* 6(1):57–58.
Luterman, D. 1995. Counseling for parents of children with auditory disorders. In *Auditory Disorders in School Children,* 3rd ed., eds. R. Roeser and M. Downs. New York: Thieme.
Luterman, D., and Kurtzer-White, E. 1999. Identifying hearing loss: Parents' needs. *American Journal of Audiology* 8:8–13.
Mahoney, G., O'Sullivan, P., and Dennebaum, J. 1990. A national study of mothers' perceptions of family-focused early intervention. *Exceptional Children* 14:133–46.
Martin, F., George, K., O'Neal, J., and Daly, J. 1987. Audiologists' and parents' attitudes regarding counseling of families of hearing-impaired children. *Asha* 29(2):27–33.
Martin, F. N., Krall, L., and O'Neal, J. 1989. The diagnosis of acquired hearing loss: Patient reactions. *ASHA* 31:47–50.
McCarthy, P., Culpepper, B., and Lucks, L. 1986. Variability in counseling experiences and training among ESB-accredited programs. *Asha* 28:49–52.
Oyler, R. F., and Matkin, N. D. 1987. National Survey of Educational preparation in pediatric audiology ASHA 29:27–33.
Roush, J. (in press) After the Screening. *The Hearing Journa*l.
Roush, J., Harrison, M., and Palsha, S. 1991. Family-centered early intervention: Professionals' perceptions. *American Annals of the Deaf* 136(4):360–6.
Roush, J., Harrison, M., Palsha, S., and Davidson, D. 1992. A national survey of educational preparation programs for early intervention specialists. *American Annals of the Deaf* 137(5):425–30.
Roush, J., and Matkin, N., Eds. 1994. *Infants and Toddlers with Hearing Loss: Family-Centered Assessment and Intervention.* Timonium, MD: York Press.
Roush, J. (DATE) Implementing parent-infant services: Advice from families. In *A Sound Foundation Through Early Amplification,* ed. R. Seewald. Phonak, AG.
Seewald, R. C., Cornelisse, L. E., Ramji, K. V., Sinclair, S. T., Moodie, K. S., and Jamieson, D. G. 1997. DSL v4.1 for Windows: A software implementation of the desired sensation level (DSLi/o) method for fitting linear gain and wide dynamic range compression hearing instruments. London, Ontario, Canada: Hearing Healthcare Research Unit, University of Western Ontario.
Simeonsson, R., Huntington, G., Sturtz-McMillen, J., Haugh-Dodds, A., Halperin, D., and Zipper, I. 1996. Services for young children and families: Evaluating intervention cycles. *Infants and Young Children* 9(2):31–42.
Sjoblad, S. (YEAR). Reactions of parents to the initial fitting of acoustic amplification in infants and young children: A national study. Master's Thesis, University of North Carolina at Chapel Hill.
Trivette, C., Dunst, C., Boyd, K., and Hamby, D. 1995. Family-oriented program models, helpgiving practices, and parental control appraisals. *Exceptional Children* 62:237–48.
Uzcategui, A., and Yoshinaga-Itano, C. (YEAR). Parents' reactions to newborn hearing screening. *Audiology Today.*
Watkin, P., Baldwin, M., Dixon, R, and Beckman, A 1998. Maternal anxiety and attitudes to universal neonatal hearing screening. *British Journal of Audiology* 32:27–37.
Yoshinaga-Itano, C., Sedey, A., Coulter, D. K., and Mehl, A. L. 1998. Language of early and later identified children with hearing loss. *Pediatrics* 102:1161–71.

Chapter ▪ 5

Current Issues in Pediatric Hearing Aid Fitting

Richard C. Seewald

My work with hearing-impaired children began in the early 1970s. The decisions I had to make at that time regarding which technology to apply were relatively straightforward. Would I fit body-worn or ear level instruments? Would I fit one ear or two? These decisions were made primarily on the basis of the child's age and the presumed degree of hearing loss in each ear. Infants (the few I saw) and toddlers with severe to profound hearing loss all received body-worn instruments. Possibly the most difficult decision I faced was in choosing among three button-type receivers (wide-band / low output; narrow-band / high output; and something in between called "standard" or "normal"). Fortunately no one ever asked me to describe the scientific principles upon which my choices were based. At that time, a complete analysis of hearing aid performance consisted of speaking into the aid at a reduced volume control wheel setting, and making a judgement about the quality of amplified sound. We did not have an electroacoustic analysis system to measure performance directly. Finally, an aided audiogram would be obtained to document benefit from amplification—and that was that.

Some of the children I fitted during those early years benefitted greatly from use of their hearing aids. Some of the children benefitted somewhat, and some did not appear to benefit at all. I had always suspected that some in the latter group wore their hearing aids only when they came to see me for their annual evaluation—it was not difficult to identify hearing aids in mint condition. However, some in the latter group did not pretend. They had discontinued their use of hearing aids for lack of any self-perceived benefit and boldly told me so. There was nothing else to offer from the "Technology Department"—it was either hearing aids or no hearing aids. The complete range of assistive technology options had been explored.

By the mid-1970s, FM "auditory trainers" had become available—large body-worn units with yet another set of button-type receivers. These systems were viewed more as educational devices than as personal amplification systems. Consequently audiologists rarely participated directly in the "selection and fitting process," such as it was. In the location where I was working, FM auditory trainers were "fitted" by the manufacturer's representative. The approach to selection and fitting of FM auditory trainers employed by these individuals can best be described as "one size fits all."

I recall one child in particular whom I had fitted with an ear level hearing aid on her right ear only. She had a severe sensorineural hearing loss in the right ear with no measurable hearing in the left. During one visit to the clinic, the mother announced that her child was now wearing an "auditory trainer" at school. Further enquiry revealed that the FM auditory trainer had been fitted by the manufacturer's representative to the child's left ear. Reportedly the advantage of this "creative arrangement" was that the child could wear both her own hearing aid and the FM auditory trainer simultaneously. No doubt, this representative had visions of himself with the Nobel Prize in hand! Unfortunately, the FM auditory trainer that was fitted to this child's "dead ear" was nothing more than an expensive illusion, as it often was in those days.

In view of the relative complexity of modern technology, the point of this story may be as relevant today as it was 25 years ago. Specifically, the availability of a given "advanced technology" does not necessarily ensure greater benefit to the child. Without informed application and continual support, the potential benefits of any "cutting-edge," "CD quality," "high-end" assistive hearing technology cannot be realized.

CURRENT ISSUES IN HEARING AID FITTING

Early Identification of Hearing Loss does not Ensure Early and Appropriate Intervention with Amplification

Those who have been around for the past 30 years or so have witnessed "on again / off again" efforts to identify hearing impairment in early infancy. My own B.Sc. Research Project (Carlin, Seewald, and Wood 1969) was designed to evaluate an innovative newborn infant hearing protocol that had just been reported by Downs and Sterrit in 1967. In that study, we "tested" the hearing of 100 neonates using a Vicon Apriton portable audiometer. The audiometer had a hand-held loudspeaker capable of producing high-level broad- and narrow-band sounds. We presented narrow-band sound of 90 decibels SPL to each newborn and watched for a "response"—eye blink, cessation of sucking, whatever.

Since the days of the "baby blasters" there have been numerous developments in newborn and infant hearing screening procedures including the "ABCDs" of the newborn nursery (high-risk registers), Crib-o-Grams, auditory brainstem response (ABR) hearing screening systems, and, most recently, otoacoustic emission (OAE) test systems. Direct evidence to support universal newborn hearing screening programs was never really there—it just seemed like the right thing to do. The "earlier the better" premise has been enough to keep the early identification wheels turning for over 30 years. Implicit in the arguments for early identification is the assumption that early identification of hearing impairment leads directly to effective treatment including the timely application of appropriate hearing technology. Some recent data lead some of us to question the validity of this assumption.

Arehart et al. (1998), from the Marion Downs National Center for Infant Hearing, have recently reported the results of a comprehensive survey carried out in 16 states that have implemented universal newborn infant hearing screening programs. This survey investigated the coordination and characteristics of universal newborn hearing screening, audiologic assessment, and intervention programs. Of particular concern is the consistent lag time that emerges from the data between the newborn hearing screening and the intervention, including the fitting of amplification. Specifically, 45% of the sites reported that, for infants identified through the universal hearing screening programs, the average initial diagnostic evaluation occurred within the first six months of life. Further, 33% of the sites reported the average age of confirmation of hearing loss was within the first six months of life. However, only 16% reported that the average age at which children were fitted with amplification was within the first six months of life. For over half of the sites (57%), the average age at which intervention was initiated was between 12 and 18 months of age. Thus, for most, the early identification of hearing impairment did not lead directly to early intervention—a disappointing finding. The substantial delay in treatment with amplification observed in this study has been documented by others (e.g., Harrison and Roush 1996).

There are many known and hypothesized factors that can delay the timely intervention with assistive hearing technologies in infants and young children (Harrison and Roush 1996). Some of these factors are under the direct control of hearing health care professionals—others are not. One factor that we can resolve emerges from the data reported by Arehart et al. (1998). Several items were included in their questionnaire to determine the type of procedures that the pediatric audiologists used in fitting of amplification with infants and young children. It was determined that sound field aided threshold behavioral testing was used by the majority of reporting sites. As Arehart et al. observe, this finding is "interesting" in light of the fact that valid behavioral threshold data are difficult, if not impossible, to obtain with infants under the age of approximately 6 to 7 months. They conclude therefore that sites that rely on behavioral audiometric data to fit hearing aids will delay intervention with amplification until the infant (young child, by the time they get it) can perform reliably on behavioral audiometric measures. Alternatives to this conventional behavioral audiometric approach to hearing aid fitting that have been developed specifically for application with infants and young children do exist (Seewald et al. 1996; Stelmachowicz, Kalberer, and Lewis 1996; Seewald et al. 1999).

Hedley-Williams, Tharpe, and Bess (1996) reported the findings of a nationwide survey designed to identify and describe current hearing aid fitting practices used by pediatric audiologists in the United States. The survey specifically explored the selection, fitting, and verification practices commonly used as well as the types of amplification devices recommended. On the basis of their findings, these researchers concluded that few pediatric audiologists in the United States use any systematic approach for selecting and fitting amplification for infants and young children, and many do not use current fitting technologies in the fitting process—that is, they identify them early, fit them late, and fit them (eventually) using procedures that are largely outdated. Those who are interested in learning about contemporary amplification fitting procedures designed specifically for application with infants and young children are referred to the *Position Statement on Amplification for Infants and Children with Hearing Loss* (1996) and to Seewald (2000).

The survey data discussed within this section indicate an urgent need to improve the delivery of intervention through hearing aid fitting and other means before any of the potential advantages of early identification can be realized. This is something that hearing health care professionals can do something about. As I have noted elsewhere (Seewald 1995):

> Regardless of the specific procedures that are applied or the general structure that is associated with the identification program; regardless of the specific device with which a child has been fitted; effective habilitation must be universally accessible to all infants and children and their families. From the consumers' perspective, the identification of a problem without (immediate) access to effective treatment is simply an empty promise. (p. 67)

Which Gizmo for Which Child?: Matching Technology to the Needs of Children

The choice I had to make in the early 1970s between the Goldentone 5000 and the Notone 03 did not challenge my decision-making abilities to any great extent. For the most part, a hearing aid was a hearing aid. Technology options were relatively limited and, consequently, so were the opportunities available to children with hearing loss. Most aids provided only linear gain (i.e., the same amount of amplification regardless of the level of the input signal) and a relatively simple form of output limiting (i.e., peak clipping). This is no longer the case. I have provided a list of many of the hearing aid options that are available for application with children today in figure 1. The list seems to grow with each passing day—and, unfortunately, so too does the complexity of the hearing aid selection and fitting process.

This new and ever-growing array of hearing aid technology brings with it new challenges to hearing health care professionals who work routinely with infants and young children. What we know is that there is no one technology that is best suited for all children. What we do not always know is which specific assistive hearing technology is best suited to the characteristics and needs of each child we work with. There are several reasons for this.

First, developments in technology outpace research. I am keenly aware of this particular problem because of the contract research I do in collaboration with industry. Over the past several years, we have been asked by hearing aid manufacturers to evaluate the benefits derived from a new technology. By the time the research process has

Linear amplification with peak clipping

Linear amplification with output compression limiting

Input compression amplification (single band):

- adjustable compression ratio
- adjustable compression kneepoint
- fixed-ratio/variable-ratio compression

Two-channel hearing aids

compression amplification in each band

compression amplification in one band/linear amplification in the other

Three (or more) channel hearing aids

Direction/multi-microphone technologies

Digitally programmable hearing aids (1, 2. 3, and more programmable memories)

Digital signal processing (DSP) hearing aids

Figure 1. Amplification options available in modern hearing aids.

reached completion, the manufacturer has already introduced the new "gizmo" onto the market. In most cases, research on the appropriate application of a given technology lags well behind development. Consequently, research findings are often not available to support the application of a given technology.

A second problem relates to the capabilities of the target population. Although not impossible (Osberger et al. 1997), it is extremely difficult to obtain valid performance measures with infants and young children. I know of very few 6-month-old infants, for example, who will sit happily for an hour of speech perception testing or who will offer a detailed description of their subjective impressions of amplified sound. Assessing the relative benefit of assistive hearing technologies in infants and young children with hearing loss is not a trivial problem, and it cannot always be assumed that data collected from adults can be used directly in pediatric applications—infants and young children are not just little adults.

Finally, from a research perspective, we are dealing with an enormously complex problem (many variables to be studied and many to be controlled). Consider, for example, all of the amplification options shown in figure 1 that are related to hearing aids. Of course all of these various hearing characteristics must be studied as they interact with a potentially large number of child characteristics. As one considers the complexity associated with this problem, it is easy to understand why many questions remain unanswered.

One area in which debate is beginning to heat up relates to the increasing trend to implant children with more residual hearing and at younger ages. Issues that are beginning to emerge from this debate are both interesting and important to all concerned. Until recently, the criteria for providing children with implants were relatively straightforward and precisely stated. To be considered as a candidate for a cochlear implant, the old rules stated that a child:

1. Must be at least 24 months of age;
2. Have a profound sensorineural hearing loss in both ears;
3. Receive little or no documented benefit from conventional acoustic amplification;
4. Have no medical contraindications for surgical implantation;
5. Be enrolled in an educational program that emphasizes the development of auditory skills; and
6. Have a family that is highly motivated and realistic in their expectations for the implant.

Overtime these "rules," largely imposed by the FDA, have been relaxed somewhat. Issues in childhood deafness are rarely if ever "black and white," although they are sometimes presented as such.

No doubt, doing away with the old hard and fast rules for implanting children is appropriate and will lead to providing many profoundly deaf children with earlier access to auditory input (Osberger 1997). There is, however, one related issue that has always been of concern to me—one that will become more important in the days ahead as the age and hearing level criteria for implantation in children are relaxed further.

In the past, it has been necessary to demonstrate, through formal measures, that children could not benefit from hearing aids before being considered for implantation. The statement went something like this: "Appropriately fitted hearing aids must be used (for some stated period of time) before determining implant candidacy." To my knowledge, few (if any) have ever questioned what is meant by this statement. Certainly it sounds reasonable and appropriately cautious.

The concern I have is that, as a field, we have yet to agree on an operational definition of "appropriately fitted hearing aids." Let's revisit the survey findings of Hedley-Williams et al. (1996). Recall that these researchers concluded that few pediatric audiologists in the United States use any systematic approach for selecting and fitting amplification for infants and young children and many do not use current fitting technologies in the fitting process. A careful examination of the Hedley-Williams data suggests that there is wide practice variation in pediatric hearing aid fitting (many clinicians doing the same thing differently). Consequently, the same child could be seen by five different audiologists and receive five different fittings. Would all five fittings be "appropriate" for this child? Would all five fittings provide the child with an equivalent degree of benefit? Perhaps, but perhaps not. It is often difficult to determine which of the available assistive hearing technologies is best suited to the needs and characteristics of a child even under the best conditions. Consequently, it is not helpful to anyone (most of all the child) to perform the all important hearing aid trial with a fitting that is sufficiently off the mark so as to "produce" a good implant candidate.

Reason for concern regarding the adequacy of pediatric hearing aid fitting practices is supported by some data reported by Chute (1997). In this study, a total of 14 cochlear implant centers in the United States, representing more than 600 children who had received implants, responded to a questionnaire concerning practices in training, hearing aid fitting, and follow up. Chute reports that, on average, 17% of the children represented in this survey required changes in their hearing aid fittings before implantation would be considered. Further, she reports that the percentage of children who required changes in their fittings varied widely across the centers with some reporting fitting modifications in more than 50% of their caseload!

Despite the findings reported by Chute (1997), I am particularly encouraged by the recent statement made by a group of individuals (Langman et al. 1996) who work in the implant field. This group has recommended that cochlear implant centers must have expertise "in applying a myriad of hearing aid technologies to profoundly deaf children . . . if appropriate recommendations are to be made." Further, Langman et al. have recommended that audiologists who work in implant centers should have the knowledge and experience to select, adjust, and evaluate powerful analog and digitally programmable hearing aids, as well as frequency transposition aids. Of course, these requirements should apply to audiologists in all work settings, who service infants, young children, and their families.

In summary, the range of assistive hearing technologies has expanded tremendously over the past 25 years or so. As both the number and the quality of technological options have grown, so too have the opportunities for children with hearing loss. Ideally, the assistive hearing technology (or combination of technologies) selected provides the child with the greatest opportunity to use his or her auditory capacity in everyday learning. There is no "best" technology for all children with hearing loss. The goal in applying technology always transcends the specific means (technology) to achieving the desired outcome. Fortunately, recent developments provide an impressive array of assistive hearing technologies that can be selected to achieve our ultimate goal of intervening with each child. However, issues that have been raised in this paper suggest that the task of improving the quality of pediatric hearing aid fitting is one the entire field needs to embrace. After all, consequences of the decisions that are made on the basis of the success or failure of the hearing aid fitting will be with the child forever.

ACKNOWLEDGMENT

Preparation of the chapter was supported by funding to the Hearing Team of the Ontario Rehabilitation Technology Consortium, Ontario Ministry of Health.

REFERENCES

Arehart, K. H., Yoshinaga-Itano, C., Thompson, V., Gabbard, S. A., and Brown, A. S. 1998, in press. State of the states: The status of universal newborn hearing identification and intervention systems in 16 states. *American Journal of Audiology*.

Carlin, T. W., Seewald, R. C., and Wood, H. 1969. Neurological implications of responses of neonates to auditory stimuli. *The Guthrie Clinic Bulletin* 38(4):189–93.

Chute, P. M. 1997. Timing and trails of hearing aids and assistive devices. *Otolaryngology—Head and Neck Surgery* 117(3):208–13.
Harrison, M., and Roush, J. 1996. Age of suspicion, identification, and intervention for infants and young children with hearing loss: A national survey. *Ear and Hearing* 17(1):55–62.
Hedley-Williams, A., Tharpe, A. M., and Bess, F. H. 1996. Fitting hearing aids in the pediatric population: A survey of practice procedures. In *Amplification for Children with Auditory Deficits*, eds. F. H. Bess, J. S. Gravel, and A. M. Tharpe. Nashville, TN: Bill Wilkerson Center Press.
Langman, A. W., Quigley, S. M., and Souliere, C. R. 1996. Cochlear implants in children. *Pediatric Otolaryngology* 43(6):1217–31.
Osberger, M. J. 1997. Cochlear implantation in children under the age of two years: Candidacy considerations. *Otolaryngology—Head and Neck Surgery* 117(3):145–9.
Osberger, M. J., Geier, L., Zimmerman-Phillips, S., and Barker, M. J. 1997. Use of parent-report scale to assess benefit in children given the Clarion cochlear implant. *The American Journal of Otology* 18(suppl):S79–S80
Seewald, R. C. 1995. Universal habilitation. *American Journal of Audiology* 4:5.
Seewald, R. C. (Ed.) 2000. A sound foundation through early amplification: Proceedings of an International Conference. Stafa Switzerland: Phonak AG.
Seewald, R C., Moodie, K. S., Sinclair, S. T., and Cornelisse, L. E. 1996. Traditional and theoretical approaches to selecting amplification for infants and young children. In *Amplification for Children with Auditory Deficits*, eds. F. H. Bess, J. S. Gravel, and A. M. Tharpe. Nashville, TN: Bill Wilkerson Center Press.
Seewald, R. C., Moodie, K. S, Sinclair, S. T., and Scollie, S. D. 1999. Predictive validity of a procedure for pediatric hearing instrument fitting. *American Journal of Audiology* 8(2):143–52.
Stelmachowicz, P. G., Kalberer, A., and Lewis, D. E. 1996. Situational hearing aid response profile (SHARP). In *Amplification for Children with Auditory Deficits*, eds. F. H. Bess, J. S. Gravel, and A. M. Tharpe. Nashville, TN: Bill Wilkerson Center Press.
The Pediatric Working Group of the Conference on Amplification for Children With Auditory Deficits 1996. Amplification for infants and children with hearing loss. *American Journal of Audiology* 5(1):53–68.

Chapter ▪ 6

Assistive Listening Technology for Infants and Young Children with Hearing Loss

Jane R. Madell

Appropriate amplification is critical for providing auditory access to children with impaired hearing. Unfortunately, amplification alone is frequently not sufficient. Even when appropriate amplification is available, many, if not most, infants and young children with severe and profound hearing loss will not be able to hear in situations in which the acoustic signal is compromised, such as when the talker is more than a few feet away, when there is competing noise, when the signal is distorted, when the speaker is not facing the child, or when the child is on the telephone.

It has long been assumed that if children had good enough language skills they could compensate for the inability to hear. Good language will enable them to "guess" at what is being said, and to fill in missing pieces; but if the material is unfamiliar (such as when learning new material in school), a child cannot "guess." Although it is true that the better a child's language skills are, the better they communicate, it is also true that even above-age language skills will not permit a child to hear what they cannot hear. It is also clear that the better hearing a child has, the easier it is for the child to learn verbal language. Although we cannot control the degree of hearing loss, we can maximize auditory access by using appropriately fitted hearing aids, and by using assistive technology to enhance the auditory signal. Assistive technology can expand the use of hearing aids and cochlear implants by providing infants and young children with access to auditory information that would not otherwise be available.

There are several goals related to the use of assistive technology in young children.

Goal 1: To improve auditory access and communication access. Hearing aids work well when the speaker and person with impaired hearing are within three feet of each other and when there is no competing noise. Unfortunately, this ideal listening condition is almost never available. Although it has long been recognized that classrooms are noisy places that require assistive technology, it has taken a much longer time to recognize that, for a person with impaired hearing, almost every setting is noisy. If we believe that it is important for children with impaired hearing to hear in all settings, we need to assess all the acoustic environments in which children spend time.

Homes and cars are extremely noisy places. If children are going to learn to use audition to develop language they must be surrounded by meaningful sound, and especially by speech. Although this may be relatively easy to accomplish for a child with a moderate hearing loss, it is not easy to accomplish for a child with a severe to profound hearing loss. To optimize access to audition, assistive technology is essential.

Goal 2: To improve access to spoken language. Children with hearing loss have more difficulty hearing in the presence of competing noise than do normally hearing children. During any time when children are learning language, they need to hear it. Optimizing audition will increase access to language. This can be most easily accomplished with the use of assistive technology.

Goal 3: To facilitate academic learning through audition. Classrooms are auditory learning environments. At least 45% of the school day is spent in listening activities (Gordon-Langbein and Metzinger 2000). The more children can hear, the easier it is for them to learn. While it is obvious that children need to hear the teacher, they also need to hear other students. Much classroom learning involves discussion—even in kindergarten. Teachers ask questions and children suggest answers. The way a teacher responds to each child's comments will provide information that is useful to other children in the class. If a hearing impaired child hears the teacher's question, but does not hear another child's answer, she or he will not learn from the discussion. If, with the use of assistive technology and modification of teaching techniques, the child can hear both the teacher and the student, the child will have significantly improved academic learning.

Goal 4: To facilitate socialization. One of the biggest difficulties children with hearing loss face is with socialization. Communication is critical for socialization. We need to hear on the playground, on the soccer field, around the snack table, and in the block corner. Assistive technology, correctly used, can improve communication in these areas. Hearing impaired children report that they have become more capable and better liked team players with FM systems because they can hear a coach's directions that were unavailable to them without assistive technology.

Goal 5: To facilitate information access and incidental learning. If everything that a child learns has to be directly taught, much information will be missing from a child's general knowledge. We have all had the experience of normal hearing children "overhearing" conversations they were not meant to hear. Although this is sometimes annoying to adults, it is critical for developing knowledge. Hearing aids alone will not permit enough auditory access for a child with a severe or profound hearing loss to maximize the use of incidental learning. Assistive technology can provide access to improve incidental learning.

Goal 6: To improve safety. Safety is a concern for all children with impaired hearing. The more severe the hearing loss, the more of a concern it becomes. Assistive technology can permit children to hear fire and smoke alarms, to know when someone is at the door, to know when the phone is ringing, and to hear a car coming down the street. It can provide a child and parent with comfort and security.

FACTORS THAT INFLUENCE INFANT/CHILD COMMUNICATION

Distance

Several factors affect infant/child communication. An uncontrollable factor is the degree of hearing loss. There are, however, several environmental factors that can be controlled, and which, if controlled, will improve communication. The first is distance between the speaker and listener. Whenever possible, the speaker should be close to the child—ideally 6 to 8 inches from the child's ear or hearing aid/cochlear implant microphone. This may be possible with an infant who is being held, but is not easy to accomplish once a child becomes mobile, either crawling or walking. Once a child is mobile, the use of a close microphone by the parent is the only way to provide consistent auditory access.

Noise

The second environmental factor that should be controlled is noise because it will affect speech perception negatively. Research by Finitzo-Heiber and Tillman (1978), Tillman, Carhart, and Olson (1970), Bess and McConnell (1981), and others has demonstrated that word recognition of hearing impaired children is significantly reduced by noise (see table I). A normally hearing child will understand 95% of words in quiet and a child with impaired hearing will understand 83%. If the signal is degraded by noise, at 0 signal-to-noise ratio, the normally hearing child will understand 60% and the hearing impaired child will understand only 39%. It is critical to control noise and to provide assistive technology to limit the negative effects of competing noise.

Some noise is easily controllable. It is easy to turn off the TV or radio when trying to communicate or to use a dishwasher only when the hearing impaired child is not in the room. Noise can be reduced by purchasing appliances that have low noise levels. Use of carpeting and rubber mats under appliances will reduce the noise of the appliances, as will carpeting in heavy traffic areas and in places where children are likely to be making noise with toys, such as the play area where blocks will be used. In areas that are not carpeted, using rubber tips on chair legs will make the movement of chairs less disturbing. Encouraging the use of rubber soled shoes or slippers will also help. Room reverberation will also affect the auditory signal negatively (see table I). The use of carpeting, drapes, and acoustical ceiling tiles will reduce room reverberation.

A final factor that can affect infant/child communication is the expectation level of the talker about the child's ability to hear. If the talker does not expect the child to be able to use audition to receive information, she or he is not likely to make any adaptations for improved communication and is not likely to try to determine if the child is able to hear. Although this is not strictly an "environmental" concern, it is definitely an issue that will affect communication. It is something that should be considered by audiologists in fitting hearing aids and by speech-language pathologists, auditory verbal therapists, and teachers of hearing impaired children when these specialists are working with families.

Sources of Noise. Homes are very noisy places. Many homes have TV and radio on much of the day, appliances are noisy and numerous; computers and computer games can also be noisy. Street traffic can be

Table I Speech Perception Scores of a Group of Normal-Hearing Children and Hard-of-Hearing Children Using Hearing Aids Under Different Reverberation Times and Speech-to-Noise Ratios.

	Normal				Hearing-Impaired			
R Time	Quite	+12	+6	0	Quite	+12	+6	0
0	95	89	80	60	83	70	60	39
0.4	93	83	71	48	74	60	52	28
1.2	77	69	54	30	45	41	27	11

Adapted from Finitzo-Hieber and Tillman (1978). Used with permission.

a significant source of noise in many homes. People are another significant source of noise. Children playing or adults talking and laughing can be very noisy and can make listening difficult. The dinner table is a very difficult listening situation because of the combination of noise from dishes and silverware, multiple people speaking, and distance from the talker.

Classroom acoustics are notoriously poor. In many schools, especially old ones, ceilings are high, windows are large, and all hard surfaces (floors, ceilings, and walls) cause sound reflection and reverberation. The movement of furniture on hard floors is noisy, as is the shuffling of papers, books, and the movement of children in their seats. Noises from the hall, street and playground, the gym, and bathrooms will contribute to the overall noise level. The noise of children talking, or even whispering, will affect communication negatively. Poor school acoustics will affect all children, not just those with impaired hearing, so acoustics should be considered in all school building plans. Listening in classrooms would be significantly improved by having low ceilings with acoustical tiling. Floors should be carpeted or covered with some kind of sound reduction tiling, preferably throughout the listening space, but at least in especially noisy areas like the block corner. To reduce the noise from the movement of chairs and desks, chair and table legs should have rubber stoppers. If stoppers are not available, discarded tennis balls can be made into stoppers. Locations of classrooms for children with hearing loss or other auditory learning problems require special consideration. They should be located on the quiet side of the building, away from noisy streets and the playground, and not near the gym or bathrooms.

Children contribute significantly to the noise of the classroom and keeping children quiet is difficult to manage. It is helpful if the classroom teacher sets a tone of general quiet, asking children not to speak out of turn.

Playgrounds, parks, or backyards create difficult listening situations, as do other open places like malls. Movie theaters, churches, or temples also present difficult listening situations because of the large open spaces with poor acoustics.

Cars create another particularly difficult listening condition for anyone with a hearing loss and the typical family exchanges that frequently take place in a car may be inaudible for a child with a hearing loss. The engine noise and either air conditioning or noise coming in from open windows make for extremely noisy conditions. A hearing impaired child is frequently seated in the back seat and cannot see the face of the parent who is speaking, making it impossible to speechread and further decreasing access to conversation. It should not be surprising that parents frequently report that children remove their hearing aids in the car. For children who use assistive listening devices, the inability to communicate in the car must be very frustrating.

TYPES OF ASSISTIVE LISTENING SYSTEMS

There are many different types of assistive listening systems. Each has an important place and, when appropriately used, can make a significant difference in a child's life.

Hearing aids

Hearing aids are the first assistive device. A detailed discussion is beyond the scope of this chapter. A brief description of hearing aid concerns follows. For further information on hearing aids see Seewald, in this text (Chapter 5; Lewis 2000; Madell 1998; and Kuk 2000).

There are many considerations in selecting appropriate amplification. The primary purpose of amplification is to provide access to speech information. Therefore, the first goal is to select amplification that brings amplified hearing into the range of conversational speech. This is not always an easy task, especially for children with severe and profound hearing loss. Although many hearing aids provide access to low frequency stimuli, access to high frequency stimuli is much more difficult to obtain for children who have significant hearing losses in this range. Inability to hear high frequencies reduces access to a great deal of information including perception of /s/, /z/, /sh/ and pluralization and possession. Some of this problem can be remedied by very careful selection of hearing aids, earmolds, and use of close microphones (most commonly with an FM system).

Hearing aid styles

Hearing aids used for children are most commonly behind-the-ear (BTE) aids. Ear level microphones provide the ability to localize and BTE hearing aids are more cosmetically acceptable than body-worn hearing aids. Although these hearing aids are appropriate for many children, they are not appropriate for all. For children with severe and profound hearing losses, it is frequently not possible to turn BTE hearing aids loud enough to provide sufficient auditory information without getting feedback. The feedback is usually so annoying to the adults in the child's environment that the hearing aid is turned down. Using a body-worn hearing aid can frequently solve this problem. The distance from the hearing aid microphone to the earmold is sufficient to reduce or eliminate feedback. Unfortunately, cosmetic concerns frequently make both audiologists and parents turn away from body-worn systems (Ross and Madell 1988). In-the-ear and in-the-canal hearing aids are not usually used with young children although they may be considered with older children and teenagers.

New technology

Until recently, only analog hearing aids were used for children. The newer programmable, digital, and multi-memory hearing aids are now used more frequently with young children. Programmable hearing aids give audiologists more control of the hearing aids setting, frequently permitting them to provide a better acoustic signal. Digital hearing aids are reported to provide clearer signals. Multi-memory hearing aids allow programming for different listening conditions enabling the user to change the setting to improve listening in quiet and noisy environments. (Young children will not be able to make use of this on their own.) Programmable, digital, and multi-memory hearing aids are just now becoming available with enough gain to meet the needs of children with profound hearing loss.

Earmolds

Earmolds are critical in maximizing acoustic information. There are many different styles, and there are earmold modifications that can make a significant acoustic difference. For example, vented earmolds can improve the auditory access for a child with good low frequency hearing, and horned earmolds can improve high frequency information. Even if a young child's ear is not sufficiently large to get a full size horn into the mold, the horn effect may provide some additional high frequency information.

Other considerations

There are a number of other considerations in selecting amplification for children. Every hearing aid should be FM compatible. There is no child who does not need an FM system in school or at home, so every hearing aid should have FM capabilities. Hearing aids selected for young children should be sturdy, have good repair records, and have a battery door that can be locked. Both hearing aids and earmolds are now available in colors. They no longer need to be boring beige or dark brown. Children who select the color of their earmolds and hearing aids may be more willing to accept that the hearing aid is part of who they are. Improving the ability to accept oneself as a hearing impaired person has many advantages.

FM systems

FM listening systems are wireless amplification systems in which the signal is transmitted to a receiver worn by the hearing impaired listener via FM radio waves from a microphone worn by the talker. FM systems are designed to reduce the negative effect of distance and competing noise on speech perception. FM systems may be integrated into hearing aids or may be separate systems that can be coupled to hearing aids, worn with earphones, or used with loudspeakers

Why do we need FM systems? The negative effect of distance on speech perception is demonstrated in figure 1. The farther the speaker is from the listener's ear or hearing aid microphone, the poorer the signal-to-noise ratio will be. By combining the information from table I, which demonstrates the negative effect of signal to noise ratio, especially for children with impaired hearing, and figure 1, which demonstrates the negative effect of distance, we can see that for a child with impaired hearing, at a distance of 6 feet, word recognition can be expected to be only 39%. At 12 feet, when the signal-to-noise ratio will be –6 decibels, we can expect that it will be even poorer. On the other hand, at a distance of 4.5 to 9 inches, the signal-to-noise ratio will be +24 to +18 decibels which will provide for maximum speech intelligibility. Because it is not possible to eliminate the negative effects of noise or distance completely, the use of a remote close microphone is

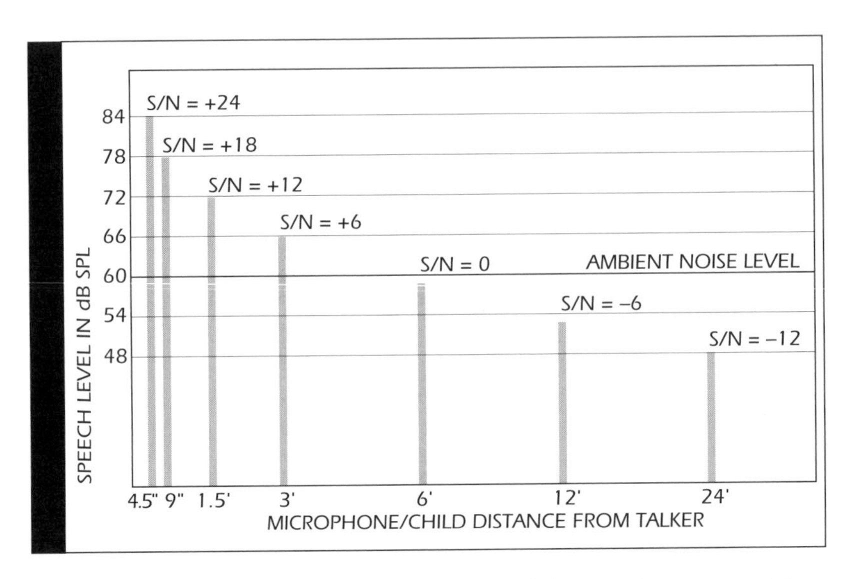

Figure 1. Speech-to-noise ratio as a function of distance in a room with an ambient noise level of 60 decibels SPL. From Ross, M. (Used with permission).

the best option for improved speech perception. Because FM systems are wireless and wearable, they permit the hearing impaired child to move freely within the home, classroom, or school building, and travel through the streets going into shops and other buildings while keeping an excellent signal-to-noise ratio. Because the close FM microphone is 4 to 6 inches from the mouth of the talker, the FM signal will be 10 to 15 decibels louder than the signal at the hearing aid microphone. This will make the parent's or teacher's voice very clear to the child. The clarity of the FM signal will be reduced somewhat when the hearing aid microphone is engaged, but the use of the hearing aid microphone will permit the child to hear him or herself and those close by. The use of the FM microphone will maintain the level of the talker's voice across distance. Research by Brackett, (1996) and others, has demonstrated that the use of an FM system as primary amplification can improve language development. It is important to note that the use of some of the new hearing aid technology that is available (such as programmable and digital hearing aids), does not preclude the need for an FM system in any critical listening situation. Although the new hearing aids may provide a better signal than analog hearing aids, they do not eliminate noise or the negative effects of distance.

Who needs an FM system? Everyone who has a hearing loss will benefit from an FM system under some circumstances. Infants and young children who are learning language through audition have a critical need for a clear auditory signal all the time. For this population, it is essential that an FM system be available to use at any time that the signal will be degraded by distance or noise. In a situation when noise and reverberation can be controlled, and where the speaker and listener are within 2 to 3 feet of each other, it may be possible to do without FM assistance. In other situations, if the child is not wearing an FM system, it is not reasonable to expect that the child will have a clear auditory signal.

All school children need FM systems. In some classes, such as pre-school, it may not be necessary to use the FM transmitter during free play periods, but an FM system is needed at any time that a teacher is communicating with a group of children. For older children, when the class is broken up into individual groups, it will be useful to have another child in the group wear the transmitter to improve auditory access for the hearing impaired child.

In addition to children with hearing loss, children with auditory processing disorders and children with auditory attention disorders will benefit from the use of an FM system. Both of these groups of children have significant difficulty hearing in the presence of competing noise and in other situations in which the speech signal is in any way degraded. FM systems which do not contain hearing aids, but only transmit the signal from the microphone, are ideal for this population.

Types of FM systems

Receiver Options. Until recently, hearing aids and FM systems were built into separate units. Hearing aids were available in body-worn and BTE styles, but FM receivers were only available in body-worn styles. Children who wore BTE hearing aids and needed both hearing aids and FM systems needed to wear two separate pieces of equipment. Technological improvements have now made it possible to get both hearing aids and FM receivers into a BTE case. These are available in a number of different formats. Some manufacturers have made hearing aids and FM receivers in one case with an antenna attached to the case (see figure 2). Other manufacturers have made an audio boot that plugs into a hearing aid and provides the FM signal (see figure 2). Very young children and children with severe and profound hearing loss may use a body-worn hearing aid/FM system that will couple to the ear with button transducers or BTE transducers. In some cases a bone vibrator may be used.

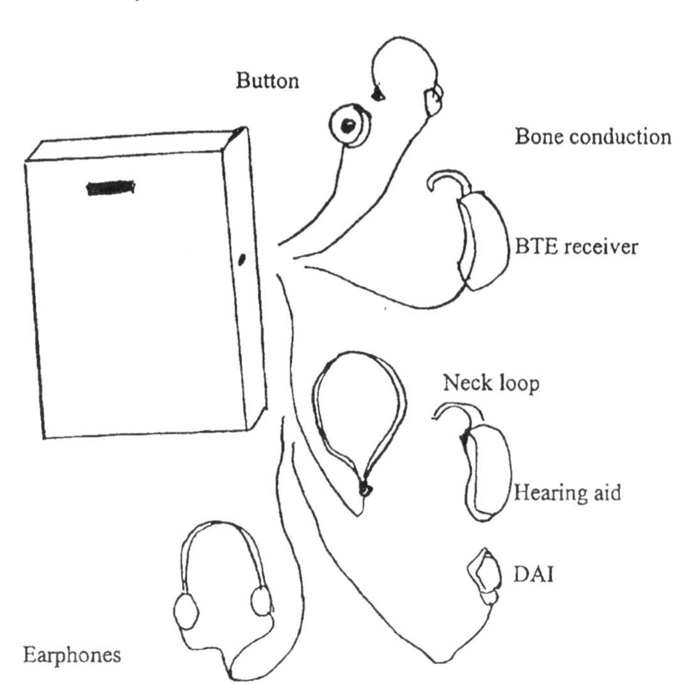

Figure 2. Body Worn FM Receiver

An FM-only system is used when a user does not need hearing aid amplification. This may be because the user has hearing aids or may be because he or she does not have a hearing loss but has an auditory processing disorder or an auditory attention disorder and is using an FM system to improve the signal-to noise ratio without adding amplification. For a child who has hearing aids, a body-worn FM system can be coupled to the hearing aids using direct audio input (DAI) by plugging an audio shoe into the hearing aid and connecting the other end of the cord into a body-worn FM system. The hearing aid may also be coupled to the FM system using a neckloop or silhouettes attached to the FM system and turning the hearing aid to the telephone setting. This requires a strong telecoil to get a good signal.

When an FM system is going to be used without a hearing aid, three types are available: BTE format, body-worn format, and soundfield format. The BTE looks like a BTE hearing aid/FM system with an antenna attached to the hearing aid case or with a self-contained FM boot attached to the BTE case (see figure 3). It has no hearing aid and simply transmits the FM signal. The body-worn system can also transmit only the FM signal and can be worn with earphones or earbuds. Two types of soundfield systems are available. A group soundfield system utilizes loudspeakers placed around the room (see figure 4). The teacher's microphone signal will be broadcast to the entire class with a gain of 6 to 9 decibels. A personal soundfield system utilizes an individual loudspeaker instead of a group loudspeaker which the child places on the desk in front of him or her.

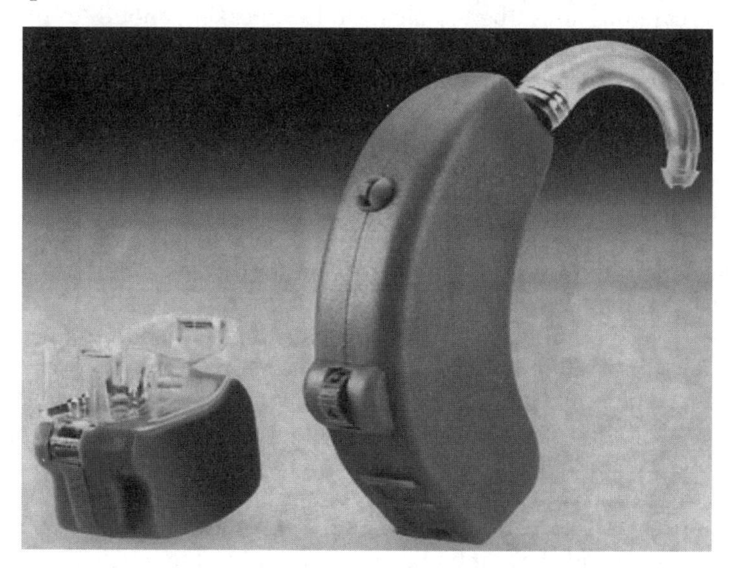

Figure 3. BTE FM Receiver. (Phonak, used with permission.)

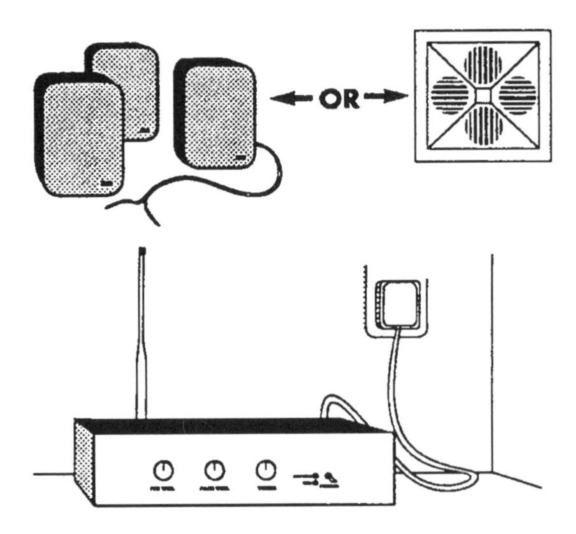

Figure 4. Soundfield FM (Phonic Ear Inc. Used with permission)

Transmitter options. There are several different transmitters (see figure 5). The most common is the clip-on microphone attached to a body-worn transmitter. This microphone is easy to use and most people find it comfortable to wear. However, if the microphone is not placed carefully it can be too far from the speaker's mouth to provide an optimal signal. The lavaliere microphone is self-contained and hangs around the neck and, because of its placement, is always located close to the mouth. The microphone that provides the best acoustic signal is the head worn (boom) microphone which is placed in front of the mouth. It provides a very clear signal but may interfere with speechreading. For group meetings or small conferences, a conference microphone will be most appropriate. The microphone has multidirectional outlets and will pick up a signal from multiple sides of the conference mike and transmit the signal to the listener's FM system.

A major problem with FM systems is the restriction to the use of only one transmitter microphone. In a classroom with two teachers, or when two parents want to use a transmitter, this can be a problem. It is possible to hook up two transmitters by using them in a daisy chain fashion. Transmitter A is worn by one person and sends a signal to the second person who is wearing receiver A which is plugged into the auxiliary jack of transmitter B. Person 2 talks into the microphone of transmitter B and the combined signal is sent to the hearing impaired person wearing receiver B. This works with only two transmitters.

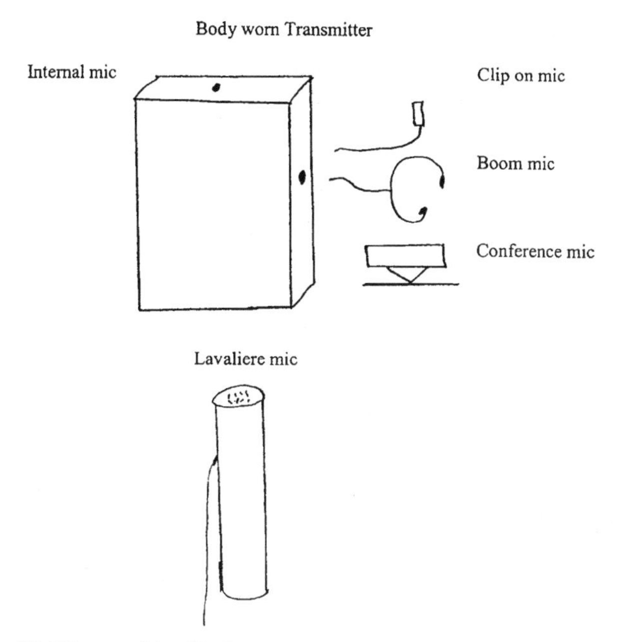

Figure 5. FM Transmitter Options

Selection of type of FM system

For children with severe to profound hearing loss, it is my view that an FM system will be needed as primary amplification because the FM will be needed most of the time. For very young children, a body-worn hearing aid/FM system may be the system of choice. It may not be possible to turn a BTE hearing aid up to the desired sound level because of the problem with feedback caused by the short distance between the BTE hearing aid microphone and the earmold; the sound transmission through the very soft cartilage of the young child's pinna; and the young child's quickly growing ears resulting in feedback from ill-fitting earmolds. This can compromise the auditory signal and be a source of frustration and annoyance to parents and clinicians alike. With the body-worn system, there is increased distance between the earmold and the hearing aid microphone, resulting in far less feedback, permitting the hearing aid to be worn at the desired setting.

Infants with less severe hearing losses may also benefit from the use of a body worn system. Before an infant is sitting upright for most of the day, it is difficult to use a BTE hearing aid because of the problems with feedback caused by the amplification pressing against the crib or stroller.

Toddlers with mild to moderate hearing losses will need FM systems less frequently because hearing aids will provide sufficient gain for them to hear in most situations. However, toddlers with moderately severe to profound hearing losses need FM systems most of the time since hearing aids alone cannot provide sufficient gain. They will not need an FM system when they are seated next to, or across the table from the person with whom they are communicating, as in a therapy session. However, as they wander around their homes, eat at the dinner table, or ride in the car, they will need an FM system. A BTE hearing aid/FM system is the easiest to use because there are no wires to catch on things and get pulled out. If the BTE system can be used at optimal gain without feedback, it should perform well. If it is not possible to use the BTE system set optimally without feedback, a body worn system should be considered.

School-aged children who have hearing aids that they use successfully, should be fitted with an FM system that couples easily to the hearing aids. Most children are more comfortable with BTE systems. However, not all hearing aids are designed to couple to a self-contained FM audio-boot. In this case, a body worn FM system with direct audio input will be the system of choice.

Older children (junior and senior high school) may wish to use in-the-ear hearing aids that are not easily coupled to FM systems. If the hearing aid has a T switch, it is possible that the hearing aid manufacturer will be able to change this to an M-T switch. If this can be done, and if the T coil is sufficiently strong, it will be possible to use the hearing aid with a neckloop attached to a body worn FM. In some cases the neckloop can be worn under the clothing making it less visible, but this may compromise the acoustic signal. If this cannot be accomplished without sacrificing the acoustic signal, it will be necessary to use a different amplification system in school. For social purposes, a BTE system would be the system of choice.

Whenever possible, a child should use the same hearing aids in school and at home, adding an FM system when needed so that the child does not have to learn to listen to different auditory signals and learn to interpret different sounds. Maximizing audition is difficult for every child with a hearing loss. Asking a child to learn to listen with two different systems that require that he or she switch auditory signals during the day, should be avoided as much as possible.

Wide band versus Narrow band. FM systems are available with wide band and narrow band transmission. Wide band transmission has higher fidelity. Narrow band transmission permits more transmission channels to be used in a small area. All children in one classroom need to use the same transmission channel or the teacher will need to wear multiple transmitters. FM systems may receive interference from outside signals including computers and cell phones. In certain areas, a narrow transmission signal may make it easier to receive a clear signal.

Coupling FM systems to cochlear implants

Yes, you still need an FM system if you have a cochlear implant. Although there is no doubt that a cochlear implant will provide significantly improved ability to hear when compared to a hearing aid, an implant does not provide normal hearing, and when the auditory signal is degraded, a cochlear implant user will have more difficulty hearing. Cochlear implants may make use of FM systems in three ways: coupled to a personal FM system, with a group soundfield FM system, or with a personal soundfield system. The personal soundfield system is currently the most popular FM choice for children with cochlear implants. These will work well if the children are always in their seats. However, if children move about their classrooms, they will need to take their loudspeakers with them and will need to carry them from room to room. They will not be able to use them for sports, gym, recreation, or lunch, and loudspeakers will be difficult to use outside of school.

A group soundfield system that places loudspeakers around the room will not provide sufficient gain to meet the need for a loud and clear acoustic signal. Coupling the implant to a personal FM system provides the best possible acoustic signal to the listener, because the signal from the transmitter microphone is going directly into the speech processor.

There are two problems, however. One is cosmetic. For most FM systems, the user will need to wear two systems (FM and implant) and this can be cumbersome. However, one manufacturer has released a small FM (about 1 inch square) that can be plugged into the accessory jack of the speech processor eliminating the need for the extra device. The second problem is more serious. Because we cannot check the quality of the FM signal on a cochlear implant user it is not possible for the audiologist or parent to tell if the FM system is working well. If the FM system works well, we will be providing the cochlear implant user with an excellent auditory signal. If not, we may be providing increased distortion. It is critical to have the correct cables for coupling the two systems. Once a child can do some speech perception testing and/or report on the quality of sound, it should not be difficult to determine if the FM system is working. However, if the child is in a noisy classroom environment, an FM system will be needed even if speech perception testing is not possible. One possibility is to test the

FM system on an older child with the same implant who can tell us if the system is working.

Appropriate use of FM systems

One concern about FM use has been the problems parents and teachers have using the FM systems appropriately. The purpose of the FM system is to improve auditory access. The FM transmitter should be worn every time a speaker is saying anything that should be heard by a hearing impaired child who is wearing a receiver. When a parent or teacher is talking with someone about something that is not important or of interest to the child, the FM system should be turned off. A young child, especially one with poor speech perception, cannot be expected to differentiate between what is important to listen to and what is not. If too much is presented that is not meaningful, the child will simply "tune out" auditory stimuli. Turning off the transmitter when it is not necessary for the child to attend will increase the probability that the child will attend when he or she hears speech through the transmitter.

Infrared Systems

Infrared systems are used in theaters, religious institutions, and other enclosed spaces and are useful for transmission of TV signals in homes. In theaters and movies, an infrared transmitter is placed near the front of the space and an infrared signal is beamed throughout the space. Individual receivers are available. Some are coupled to hearing aids through direct audio input, or using a neck loop and putting the hearing aid on the telephone setting. Others are worn like earphones. A smaller version of the infrared system is available for home use and can be plugged into the TV or radio, or a small microphone can be plugged into the transmitter and placed in front of the TV speaker to transmit TV signals. Since infrared signals are transmitted by light, the system cannot be used outside in sunlight. Because of the light sensitivity they are not good systems for use in schools, but can be useful when children go to the movies or theater.

Loop Systems

An induction loop can be placed around a room where hearing impaired children or adults meet regularly. This is frequently done by placing the induction coil in a grid under a carpet. Hearing impaired children then turn their hearing aids to the telephone coil setting and hear the information that is transmitted over the microphone. This was a very popular system for schools prior to FM use and they are still used in meeting places outside of schools. Rooms with induction loops need to be physically separated or there may be a problem with children in one room picking up signals from the next room. Another problem with these systems is related to the quality of the telecoils in many hearing aids. If the telecoil is not strong, the signal the child receives will be weak. If the hearing aid does not have an M-T switch, when the hearing aid is switched to the T position, the child will hear the teacher, but not hear anything that is being said by children close by.

Hard Wired Systems

Prior to the use of FM systems, hard wired systems were used in school programs and for speech therapy. A microphone was attached to an amplifier and children wore earphones that were also attached to the amplifier. At the time that they were popular, they provided the best signal available (superior to the hearing aids that were available) and were used for speech training. The limits of being restricted by the length of the cord from the amplifier to the earphones are obvious.

Telephone Systems

A number of different systems are available that will improve the ability of children and adults with impaired hearing to be alerted to the telephone ring and to communicate on the phone. Telephone systems are divided into two parts: alerting systems to permit the hearing impaired child to know that the phone is ringing, and communication systems to enable the hearing impaired child to communicate by phone. The ability to use the phone may not seem critical for a young child, but it is important because of its role in socialization. Children with impaired hearing need to recognize what a phone does, and if possible, learn to communicate using it.

Alerting systems. Hearing impaired children frequently do not know when the phone is ringing. The first concern is to alert them to the sound of the telephone. Alerting systems include flashing lights, loud bells or buzzers, and bed vibrators that go off when the phone rings. Children can be taught to recognize that the phone is ringing and to go to the phone to answer it.

Telephone communication. Some children will be able to learn to hear on the telephone with their hearing aids or FM systems. This may be accomplished using the telecoils of the hearing aid or by placing the speaker from the telephone handset close to the microphone of the hearing aid or FM. In both cases, it will take practice to find the placement that provides the best signal. Having an amplified telephone will frequently help. Some children with mild to moderate hearing losses may be able to hear on the phone by using an amplified telephone without hearing aids. Amplified telephone handsets are available from phone companies and portable telephone amplifiers are available from hearing aid dispensers, from stores like Radio Shack, and from mail order companies.

It is possible to couple the hearing aid or cochlear implant directly into some telephones. Some telephones have jacks, and a neckloop or direct audio input plug can be plugged in and connected to the hearing aid. Cords are available to connect hearing aids into cordless phones. Some users find speaker phones a good way to communicate because it enables them to use two ears or two hearing aids. When purchasing a phone, it is important to know if the phone is hearing aid compatible if the child is going to be using the telephone with the "T" coil of the hearing aid.

For people who cannot use audition on the telephone, telephone communication is possible using a teletypewriter (TTY). Both the listener and sender need TTYs to send and receive messages. If someone who does not have a TTY wishes to communicate with someone with a TTY, he or she can make use of relay services that are available in most states. If a telephone user who communicates using audition wants to contact someone who uses a TTY, he or she phones the relay services, the relay calls the person who uses the TTY and acts as a translator, translating the voice message into a typed message and vice-versa. Very young children will obviously have difficulty using this system since they cannot read or write.

Training to use the telephone. Many children will not be able to hear on the phone when they first try, but like any other form of listening, it can frequently be learned. A good way to start training is to have the child listen on the phone and have a parent use a cordless extension phone and stand next to the child to help translate what the child cannot hear, or repeat what is said so the child can speech-read. Initially, a very patient relative or friend can be on the phone talking to the child about familiar, pre-arranged topics. As the child's skills improve he or she can venture out and answer the phone without knowing who is on the phone or what will be discussed.

TV Systems

For children who use audition to monitor television, there are a number of different systems that can improve the ability to hear. The infrared system described above is a very useful system for many people. An FM system can also be used by hanging the transmitter microphone in front of the TV speaker, or connecting the FM system to the TV using the auxiliary jack on the FM transmitter. The child will use the FM receiver in the same way he or she does at school. A personal soundfield loudspeaker system can be placed next to the child's seat to transmit the TV signal. A direct-audio-input system can jack directly into the television and couple to the hearing aid. A radio tuned to the TV station can be placed next to the child's chair to provide a louder signal without any additional devices. Once children learn to read, they can make use of closed captioning which is available with many TV programs.

ASSISTIVE LIVING SYSTEMS

Assistive living systems provide hearing impaired children with independence, privacy, and safety. Normally hearing children use audition for much more than the ability to understand speech. They use hearing to know the phone is ringing and to speak on it, to hear the doorbell or someone knocking, to know if someone is at their bedroom door, and for such safety concerns as smoke and fire alarms, and car horns. When they are old enough, children wake themselves up with an alarm clock and chat with friends on the phone. Hearing impaired children need to do these same things. If they cannot do them with hearing aids, other systems need to be developed so that they can develop the same maturity, responsibility, and independence as their normally hearing peers. Parents and teachers of children with impaired hearing frequently neglect to provide children with access to sounds around them. Initially it is because they know the children cannot easily hear them and because learning to listen and talk seems more important. It is, however, important that hearing impaired children become included in the environment. Alerting systems are available that can let a hearing impaired person know that the door, phone, or an alarm is going off using flashing lights, a bed vibrator, or loud bells or buzzers. They can learn to identify which system is activated by recognizing differences in the rate of flashing lights, bells, buzzes, or vibrations (one, two, three; two shorts and one long). The use of an alarm system and a phone system will help both parent and child feel more secure when the child is home alone. Children can gain independence by learning to wake themselves with an alarm clock, and to have private phone conversations with whatever phone technology they require. They can have privacy by being able to tell when someone is at their bedroom door and by not requiring assistance to use the phone. (Many hearing impaired teenagers find that having an alerting system on their bedroom door gives them very valued privacy—it eliminates the door being opened without warning by parents needing to transmit a message.) It is important not to wait until children are leaving home to teach them to use assistive living technology. Even young children should use assistive systems so they can learn to do the same things their normal hearing peers are being asked to do.

MANAGING THE ACOUSTIC ENVIRONMENT

There are basically three ways to manage the acoustic environment: use of a close microphone (which we have discussed above in the section on FM systems), use of acoustical treatment to reduce noise, and modification of communication style.

Acoustical treatment of the environment

The use of acoustical treatment can significantly reduce unwanted noise. Begin by determining sources of noise. Carpeting with rubber padding will reduce the noise of footsteps, movement of chairs, and dull other sounds by reducing reverberation. Acoustical tiles on the ceiling can significantly reduce noise and reverberation. If the ceiling is high, it can be lowered, which will further reduce reverberation. The use of heavy drapes covering windows can reduce reverberation and reduce sounds from the street. In a large room like a classroom, cork or fabric bulletin boards can serve the dual purpose of providing a place to hang art and reduce reverberation by eliminating hard wall surfaces. Noise can be reduced if noisy appliances in the home, and computers and projectors in schools are placed on rubber mats to reduce vibration. Soft couches and pillows on chairs will reduce reverberation caused by sound reflection on hard surfaces.

Noise should be controlled as much as possible. Turn off TV and radio, do not run the dishwasher or washer/dryer when trying to communicate. Use place mats at the table to reduce the noise of plates and glasses.

Use of a close microphone. The use of a close microphone available in an FM system and in some other assistive devices, will reduce the negative effects of distance and competing noise. While a close microphone will not eliminate noise, it will bypass most of it making a parent's or teacher's voice sound as if the talker were standing next to the child's ear, hearing aid, or cochlear implant. If two talkers need to communicate with the child, it is possible to connect two FM systems that permits two people to use FM microphones.

If communication is taking place around a table such as at dinner or for small group work in school, it may be useful to use a conference microphone (an FM microphone placed in a stand which, when placed in the middle of a table, will pickup conversations from all directions around the table).

Modification of communication style. An important technique for managing the acoustic environment is the use of techniques to improve communication style. The speech of a person wearing the FM transmitter will be clear to the hearing impaired child. Others who are not near the FM microphone or child's hearing aid microphone will not be easy to hear. The person with the transmitter is responsible for repeating comments of others who are not using a microphone to enable the hearing impaired person to hear what they are saying.

CONCLUSION

The use of assistive technology can have a great impact on how hearing impaired children learn language and learn to become independent and responsible members of society. Families, teachers, speech pathologists, and audiologists need to be alert to children's listening environments to determine when a child is not hearing well. It is important that everyone be optimistic about what a child can learn to hear, and set up the environment for success. By providing the right equipment, expectations, and training, the opportunity for success is significantly improved.

REFERENCES

Anderson, K. 1989. *Screening Instrument for Targeting Educational Risk* (S.I.F.T.E.R). Austin, TX: PRO-ED.

Anderson, K. 1996. *Screening Instrument for Targeting Educational Risk in Preschool Children* (Preschool S.I.F.T.E.R.). Educational Audiology Association.

Benoit, R.1989. Home use of FM amplification systems during early childhood years. *Hearing Instruments* 40:8–12.

Bess, F., and McConnell, F. 1981. *Audiology, Education, and the Hearing Impaired Child.* St Louis: C. V. Mosby

Brackett, D. 1996. Developing auditory capabilities in children with severe and profound hearing loss. In *Amplification for Children with Auditory Deficits*, eds. F. H. Bess, J. S. Gravel, and A. M. Tharp. Nashville, TN: Bill Wilkerson Center Press.

Crandall, C., Smaldino, J., and Flexer, C. 1995. *Sound-Field FM Amplification: Theory and Practical Applications.* San Diego: Singular Press.

Finitzo-Hieber, T., and Tillman, T. 1978. Room acoustics effects on monosyllabic word discrimination ability for normal and hearing impaired children. *Journal of Speech and Hearing Research* 21:440–58.

Gordon-Langbein, A., and Metzinger, M. 2000. Technology in the classroom: To maximize listening and learning. *Volta Voices* Jan/Feb:10–13.

Kuk, F. 2000. Recent approaches to fitting nonlinear hearing aids. In *Audiology Treatment*, eds. M. Valente, H. Hosford-Dunn, and R. J. Roeser, Vol. II. New York: Thieme.

Lewis, D. 1991. FM systems and assistive devices: Selection and evaluation. In *Pediatric Amplification: Proceedings of the 1991 National Conference*, eds. J. A. Feigin and P. G. Stelmachowicz. Omaha, NE: Boys Town National Research Hospital.

Lewis, D. 2000. Hearing instrument selection and fitting in children. In *Audiology Treatment*, eds. M. Valente, H. Hosford-Dunn, and R. J. Roeser. New York: Thieme.

Madell, J. R. 1990. Managing classroom amplification. In *Hearing Impaired Children in the Mainstream*, ed. M. Ross. Timonium, MD: York Press.

Madell, J. R. 1992. FM systems as primary amplification for children with severe and profound hearing loss. *Ear and Hearing* 13:102–7.

Moeller, M. P., Donaghy, K. F., Beauchaine, K. L., Lewis, D. E., and Stelmachowicz, P.G. 1996. Longitudinal study of FM system use in nonacademic settings: Effects on language development. *Ear and Hearing* 17(1):28–41.

Robbins, A. M., Renshaw, J. J., and Berry, S. 1991. Evaluating meaningful auditory integration in profoundly hearing-impaired children. *American Journal of Otology* 12:144–50.

Ross, M. 1992. Room acoustics and speech perception. In *FM Auditory Training Systems: Characteristics, Selection, and Use*. Timonium, MD: York Press.

Ross, M., and Madell, J. R. 1988. *Premature Demise of Body Worn Hearing Aids*. ASHA.

Tillman, T. W., Carhart, R., Olson, W. O. 1970. Hearing aid efficiency in a competing speech situation. *Journal of Speech and Hearing Research* 13:789–811.

Chapter ▪ 7

Cochlear Implants: *Historical Overview and Current Outcomes*

Patricia M. Chute

The cochlear implant is now considered a viable treatment option for children and adults with severe to profound bilateral sensorineural hearing loss (NIH 1995). This technology has evolved over the past two decades to the degree that it can offer substantial auditory perception to its users. For young deaf children, early implants can provide a means of developing good speaking and listening skills. For more than 70% of adults who are late deafened, implants can make interactive telephone conversation possible (REF). As these devices continue to evolve, it is expected that performance will continually improve.

The team at the Cochlear Implant Center at Lenox Hill Hospital in New York has been actively involved in implantation since 1979. As of June 1, 2000, more than 489 children and adults have received various types of cochlear implants through this institution (see table I). The overall number of cochlear implant surgeries being performed worldwide each year has grown steadily as performance has improved and more centers have become involved with the technology (Niparko 2000).

A HISTORY OF COCHLEAR IMPLANTS

The first clinical attempt to stimulate the cochlea occurred in France in 1957, when Djourno and Eyries placed a gold electrode on the

Table I. Coclear Implant Center Lenox Hill Hospital

Device	Adults	Children	Total
3M/House	18	18	36
Nucleus 22	45	94	139
Clarion	39	47	86
Med El	5	3	8
Nucleus 24	54	166	220
Total	161	328	489

promontory of an adult undergoing stapes surgery under local anesthesia (Djourno and Eyrie 1957). During this procedure, the patient reported hearing a sound. It was not until the early 1960s that research related to the electrical stimulation of the cochlea was begun in the United States. The early work by House, Michelson, and Simmons occurred simultaneously in three separate laboratories in California. Although House initially used a multiple electrode array, he concentrated his efforts on a single electrode system. Michelson and Simmons focused their attention on multiple electrode arrays. Later, Schindler continued with Michelson's research. Abroad, work in the implant field was also occurring in Australia under the supervision of Clark, in Austria under Hochmaier and Burian, and in France under Chouard.

The first clinical trials of cochlear implants were performed during the 1970s in the United States under the auspices of the US Food and Drug Administration (FDA), the organization that oversees all research related to the safety and efficacy of drugs and devices. The process through which a device, like a cochlear implant, must pass before being approved for clinical use consists of several stages. The first stage is known as the experimental stage. During this phase, one or two research laboratories might investigate a device in a small sample to determine if there is reason to investigate its use in a larger population. Once the device passes from the experimental stage, the center (or manufacturer) will apply for an investigational device exemption (IDE). During this stage, other clinical centers across the United States are invited to participate in the rigorously controlled studies that are required to determine if the device is safe and effective in the larger population. In order to participate in these studies, centers must have approval from their individual Institutional Review Boards that oversee human subjects research projects. After a period of data collection, the results of these studies are presented to the FDA to determine if the device can receive pre-market approval. Once a device is pre-market approved then it can be offered to any clinical center wishing to use the device.

The concept of a clinical trial is specific to the United States. Other countries now have similar types of organizations that oversee research but none are at the level of those carried out in this country. When the early single channel implants were being assessed, there were only seven clinical centers that received an investigational device exemption from the Food and Drug Administration. The technology at this time was rudimentary. The external transmitters were held in place using a headband or eyeglasses. The speech processors were bulky and powered by two 9-volt batteries. The evaluation procedures for determining candidacy included a series of audiological and psychological tests. Because test batteries that are used today did not exist in the 1970s, much of the benefit documented was anecdotal. This created a great deal of skepticism in the medical community regarding the efficacy of the device. In 1977, Bilger and his colleagues performed an independent study of a group of adults implanted with the House device. They reported that all subjects were able to detect pure tones at 40 decibels hearing level (HL) and that many were able to detect timing and intensity cues. None of the individuals who received the implants were able to understand speech without the aid of visual cues; however, they all reported an improved quality of life.

Although there appeared to be some benefit, the bulkiness of the speech processor and the cumbersome nature of the transmission system made the technology questionable for use in children. In 1980, breakthrough technology in the form of a rare earth magnet was developed. This magnet would allow for transmission of the signal across the skin, eliminating the need for headbands and eyeglasses, thereby leading the way for the use of implants in children. This discovery changed the face of implantation and spurred increased interest in the field. At this time in the United States, the Minnesota Mining and Manufacturing Company (3M Corporation) entered the market place by providing technical support and financial backing for the House device. Years later, 3M would withdraw from the cochlear implant field and sell the rights to another implant manufacturer, Cochlear Corporation.

The clinical trials of the 3M/House device ended with the pre-market approval of the implant in 1983 for use in the adult population. By this time, clinical trials investigating other devices had begun through Cochlear Corporation, the manufacturer of the Nucleus device resulting in pre-market approval for the Nucleus 22 in adults in 1984 and for children in 1989. Simultaneously, research at the University of California, San Francisco (UCSF) and in Utah was occurring with the investigation of the Symbion (later known as the Ineraid) and the UCSF device (later known as the Clarion). The Ineraid device never received pre-market approval and was later bought by Cochlear Corporation (Niparko and Wilson 2000).

In the early 1990s a second manufacturer entered the United States market. Advanced Bionics Corporation, maker of the Clarion device, began clinical trials in adults and children and received pre-market approval for use in adults in 1996 and in children in 1997. During this same period, a third manufacturer, Med El Corporation entered the United States market with its Combi 40+ device, which is awaiting approval for children and adults. In the year 2000, there were numerous devices within these three companies that were undergoing investigation. All of them were attempts to improve the performance, the efficiency, and the cosmetic appearance of these systems.

Most recently, there has been a movement towards miniaturization of the external components. Cochlear Corporation was the first to develop successfully a clinical unit that was encased in a behind-the-ear (BTE) model. This system was part of their Nucleus 24 device that incorporated new speech processing strategies and the BTE, known as the Esprit. Additionally, a BTE system for use with the Nucleus 22 implants is now available. The Clarion device BTE, known as the Platinum BTE, scheduled to be available during the last quarter of 2000 and the Med El Tempo+BTE are presently being distributed to a small group of adult subjects.

CURRENT ISSUES IN COCHLEAR IMPLANTATION

The field of implantation has changed markedly through the years as the performance of these devices has improved. Consequently, issues regarding implantation have progressed from the viability of the device as an auditory prosthesis to changing criteria for candidate selection and its effects on education and language. Currently, there are numerous topics of interest in the implant field with respect to the changing criteria, including use of these devises in children and adults with residual hearing, the use of implants in infants, the use of these devices in children with multiple handicaps, implants for the adolescent and elderly population, and bilateral implants. Other issues surrounding implantation include the changes in technology itself, the effects that universal newborn hearing screening will have on the process, the effects on language acquisition and educational achievement, the role that managed care plays, professional training issues, and issues with Deaf Culture.

Changing Criteria in Cochlear Implantation-Residual Hearing

Historically, only individuals with profound bilateral hearing loss and no demonstrated benefit from conventional hearing aids received cochlear implant systems. As performance with these devices improved, however, there has been a movement toward the implants for children and adults with residual hearing. Numerous studies have investigated the use of implants in individuals who demonstrate some benefit from traditional amplification (Hodges, Schloffman, and Balkany 1997). The results of these studies have indicated that the cochlear implant can improve speech perception abilities in individuals with residual hearing that surpasses their performance with hearing aids. This improvement in performance has resulted in the pre-operative criteria for candidacy being changed to include individuals with some aided open set speech recognition ability on sentence material. In the most recent clinical trials, the Food and Drug Administration has approved inclusion of adults with < 50% speech recognition ability on sentence material in the implanted ear and < 60% bilaterally.

Use of Implants in Infants

As of June, 2000, the Food and Drug Administration approved the Nucleus 24 device for infants who are 12 months of age. Similar permission is being sought for the Clarion system. Also, children younger than 12 months can be implanted if it is deemed medically necessary, as in the case of the youngest child in the United States to receive a cochlear implant at 5 months of age. This child was deafened secondary to meningitis and demonstrated cochlear ossification on CT scans. The decision to implant was based on the fact that further delaying the procedure might preclude insertion of the full electrode array.

The Cochlear Implant Center at Lenox Hill Hospital has inserted the implants in 47 children (28 males and 19 females), between the ages of 11 and 24 months. The average age at diagnosis was 11.8 months with a range of 0 to 21 months. Table II displays the auditory performance of these children according to changes in speech perception categories. Because many of these children had limited linguistic competence during the very early stages of implant evaluation, to assess the perceptual abilities a series of questionnaires was developed.

Table II. Very Young Children Demographics

- 47 children receive cochlear implants
  - –28 male, 19 female
  - –Average age at diagnosis 11.8 months
    - Range 0–21 month
  - –Average, median age at implant 20 months
    - Range 10–24 months

The Infant Toddler Meaningful Auditory Integration Scale (IT-MAIS) is one of the tests that has gained popularity in evaluating infants. The results on the IT-MAIS demonstrate significant improvement at the 6- and 12-month post operative interval. These results are displayed in table III, and support the use of implants for children at very young ages. Children in this sample will continue to be monitored over time for changes in speech perception and language ability.

Children with Multiple Handicapping Conditions

The vast majority of children receiving cochlear implants has been those who do not exhibit other cognitive handicaps. There have been children implanted with non-cognitive handicaps such as Usher's Syndrome who have demonstrated good performance (Chute and Nevins 1995). Studies in Europe (Lenarz 1998) have demonstrated that there may be some utility to placing an implant in children with both cognitive and non-cognitive handicaps as long as there is proper rehabilitation and the children are young. I (2000) reported on a subset of 27 children who demonstrated a variety of handicaps that included autism, Ausberger, PDD, and low muscle tone. As a group, these children performed well with the exception of the autistic child. As the age of implantation lowers, there is a higher probability that children will be diagnosed with deafness first, and later with another type of handicap. For this reason, this subset of the cochlear implant population requires further intensive study.

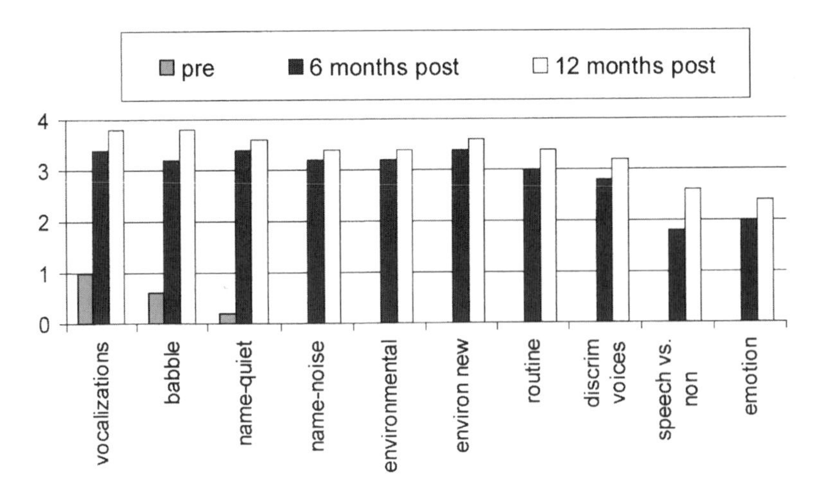

Figure 1. Average IT-MAIS

Table III. Multiply Handicapped Children Demographics

- N = 25 children
  –16 females, 9 males
- Average age at implant 3.56 years
  –Range 12 months–9.7 years
- Average duration implant use 3.61
  –Range 11 months–11 years
- Devices
  –5 Nucleus 22, 5 Clarion, 15 Nucleus 24
  –Re-implantations for 2 Clarion, 1 N22 and 1 N24

Use of Implants in Adolescents

As the cosmetic aspect of implantation has improved with the introduction of the behind-the-ear speech processor, more adolescents have begun to seek implants. This population, in general, is notorious for non-use of hearing aids and unrealistic expectations (Nevins and Chute 1995). Most adolescents do not understand the time commitment and the slow progress that occurs for this group. Instead, they often focus on the fact that it will improve their own ability to produce intelligible speech, a fact that is not true and often elusive until many years later. It is therefore critical that candidacy criteria are decided upon carefully and that guidelines for evaluation include an extensive component of counseling. The adolescents presently seeking implantation and who are considered candidates are continuous hearing aid users who are mainstreamed educationally, and who demonstrate relatively good oral skills. Those individuals who are educated in schools for the Deaf and use only a manual form of communication are not considered good implant candidates.

In a group of 24 adolescents followed at Lenox Hill Hospital in New York, 13 of the children were congenitally deaf, nine progressively deafened, and two had had meningitis. Of the congenitally deaf, six were oral (four fully mainstreamed, two partial mainstream), while seven were classified as using a signed English system (two School for the Deaf, five mainstreamed with full time sign support). The group of progressively deafened adolescents consisted of five oral children (fully mainstreamed) and four children who used sign supported English (two School for Deaf, two mainstreamed with partial support). The two children who had had meningitis had extremely different profiles. One child was oral and fully mainstreamed, and the other (partial insertion of electrode array due to ossification) was partially mainstreamed with a sign interpreter.

Performance of the overall group varied, with the majority of adolescents obtaining either open set speech recognition or consistent word recognition. This occurred for both the oral communicators and those who used a signed English system. Only one individual (partial insertion) has not progressed past pattern perception post implantation. All of the adolescents are full time CI users.

Implants in the Elderly

As performance with implants improved, a concomitant increase in individuals of all age groups seeking implants occurred. The elderly population (65 years or older) is yet another group where the number of implant recipients has grown. In a group of 38 subjects followed by the Lenox Hill Hospital Cochlear Implant Center, 20 males and 18 females ranging in age from 65.1 to 86.1 years received implants. Four subjects are now deceased. Eight of the subjects sustained a reimplantation due either to a failed internal receiver or an upgrade in technology. Subjects were implanted with either the 3M/House single channel, Nucleus 22, Nucleus 24, Clarion, or Med El device. Overall performance in this population is equivalent to the performance of average adult population with a similar trend demonstrating wide variability. It should be noted however that the poorest performers were generally the oldest recipients.

Approximately one-third of the subjects in the total group were able to use the telephone in an interactive manner. A wide range of performance was noted and dependent upon the speech processing strategy and type of device, with the poorest performers using the single channel system. Overall, if the individual is in generally good health, age should not preclude cochlear implantation in this population.

Bilateral Implants

The University of Iowa (Gantz 2000) has received FDA approval for the study of bilateral implants in the post-linguistically deafened adult population. As of February 2000, a total of nine subjects received implants in each ear. Only two subjects have been followed for one year. The remaining subjects had three month follow-up data available at the time of the report. The surgery for each of these subjects was performed on both sides at the same time. Performance improvements were noted for speech in noise with many of the patients demonstrating ceiling effects. Improvements were also noted in localization skills. Since the sample was still relatively small with a short duration of follow up, these data are considered preliminary and require a larger number of subjects to be followed for a longer period of time.

In September 2000, Cochlear Corporation announced the introduction of a clinical trial in the United States to begin the investigation of bilateral implants in both adults and children. The protocol for each of these groups is under development at the present time.

Technology Advances

There has been a series of advances in cochlear implantation over the past several years, with particular attention to the speech processing strategies, the software, and the external hardware. A wide variety of speech processing strategies is available, with each unique to a particular device. Presently, the Nucleus 24 system is capable of using strategies known as SPEAK (Spectral Peak), CIS (Continuous Interleaved Sampling), and ACE (Advanced Combined Encoder). The Clarion device supports CIS (Continuous Interleaved Sampling), PPS (Paired Pulsatile Stimulation), and SAS (Simultaneous Analog Stimulation). Med El uses strategies that are known as N of M or CIS (Wilson 2000).

Recently, a number of hardware innovations have been developed with respect to the internal electrode array. Cochlear Corporation, manufacturer of the Nucleus 24 device, has introduced a new system called the Contour that uses a pre-coiled electrode (Cochlear Corporation 2000). The rationale for using a pre-coiled system is to attempt to stimulate the residual neural elements more efficiently, thereby using less power and possibly obtaining more discrete stimulation. With a similar purpose in mind, Advanced Bionics Corporation, manufacturer of the Clarion system, has introduced a new electrode known as the Hi Focus that uses a positioner to situate the electrode closer to the modiolar region (REF). Finally, Med El has developed both a split electrode array and a compressed array to use in cochleae that may be ossified.

Other hardware innovations include the introduction of new external speech processors and headset systems. The Nucleus 24 and the Nucleus 22 support behind-the-ear models as well as the traditional body worn units. Advanced Bionics has introduced their platinum series that includes a new smaller body worn processor, with plans for a behind-the-ear processor scheduled for late 2000. Med El has introduced the Tempo+ behind-the-ear speech processing system in a selected group of adult users.

Software innovations other than those related to the speech processing strategies include the techniques known as Neural Response Telemetry (NRT) (Cochlear Corporation 2000). Neural Response Telemetry is only available in the Nucleus 24 at the present time. Neural Response Telemetry measures the action potential at each implanted electrode. This information can be used to confirm implant function, assist in the estimation of threshold and comfort levels during programming, and provide an objective assessment measure over time. Some future applications of NRT might include a method of selecting optimal sites of stimulation, optimal rates of stimulation, and optimal stimulation mode.

Effects of Universal Newborn Hearing Screening

As of June, 2000, universal newborn hearing screening was mandated in 24 out of 50 states. The result of these screenings will automatically increase the number of children who will be identified with hearing loss at earlier ages. This will require the addition of more speech and hearing professionals in our field who are trained in early childhood hearing loss and its effects. Although the majority of these children will be hard of hearing, the number diagnosed as deaf may seek implants at earlier ages. The ramifications of early implantation will have a profound effect on implantation, language acquisition, education, and the Deaf Community.

Language/Educational Outcomes

Robbins et al. (1999) and Bollard et al. (1999) have demonstrated the effects of cochlear implants on the language development of young children. Overall, the group of children with implants performed better on tests of receptive and expressive language than deaf children without implants. Typically, the gap in language abilities between deaf and hearing children increases as the children get older. Although the children with implants did not, as a group, completely close the language gap that was present at the time of the implant, this gap did not show any increase over time. Since these studies have only been recently performed, it is believed that this gap will eventually decrease.

Educationally, children with implants are entering the mainstream earlier, often within 3 to 4 years of implantation (Nevins and Chute 1995). These children have an array of support services once they are in the mainstream that might include sign language interpreters, cued speech transliterators, aides, or note takers. As the age of implant decreases, more children will begin their education in regular classrooms. Once in the mainstream children must be carefully monitored to insure success.

Reimbursement Issues and Professional Training

At the present time, managed care, private insurers, Medicare, and in some states, Medicaid, reimburse for cochlear implantation. In some cases, managed care plans may restrict access to certain centers or surgeons, thereby limiting the patients' choices. Since managed care plans consider cost containment a priority, it is unclear what effect this will have in the long term.

As noted previously, with the increased numbers of children who will be diagnosed through universal newborn hearing screening, there will be a much higher demand for professionals in the field. Reimbursement issues, therefore, are critical for personnel who are required to treat this population effectively. Additionally, training new members of the field for a specialty in cochlear implantation will require time. Institutions of higher education may not be prepared to meet the demand in a timely manner.

Deaf Culture and Cochlear Implants

The evolution of cochlear implants occurred during a period in the United States when the "Deaf President Now" movement had reached its peak. In the late 1980s there was national media attention drawn to the uprising at Gallaudet University and the political agenda of the Deaf was finally realized. Simultaneously, the cochlear implant received approval for use in children, thereby documenting the long-term benefits and supporting a growing availability. Although the evolution in technology marked it as a viable device, the skepticism of the Deaf Community was and still remains a reaction to previous impractical technologies.

The National Association for the Deaf position statement on implants in children at that time was directly opposed to its use in the pediatric population. Today this position statement is under review to address the movement that has occurred in the implant field. What role schools for the Deaf will play, along with the role of Deaf personnel, remains to be seen. As more children are receiving implants, more state schools for the Deaf are beginning to incorporate programs that can address these children's hearing and speech needs. It will most likely take a generation of implant users to determine the impact of implant technology on building the bridge between the hearing and Deaf community.

The Future

Cochlear implant technology has evolved from the early days when speech processors functioned with only a single electrode and delivered a crude signal to assist in speech-reading and environmental sound detection. The present day systems are capable of delivering sound to severe and profoundly deaf adults and children so that adults can now use the telephone interactively and children can develop near normal speaking and listening skills.

The next generation of implants almost certainly will be smaller and more efficient, with better speech processing strategies. Eventually, these devices will become fully implantable. In the interim, there may also be devices that use a hybrid hearing aid/cochlear implant system. Finally, the field of hair cell regeneration and genetic coding may someday eliminate deafness from the population. What impact this will have on Deaf Culture is unknown.

What is known, is that technology usually has a forward momentum that seldom returns to the status quo. The Deaf Community and Culture will not disappear as long as there are individuals who value its language and mores. The cochlear implant and future technologies can co-exist with this Community as long as we remain aware of the contributions that each produces.

REFERENCES

Advanced Bionics Corporation. 2000. Investigational Device Exemption G990146. The investigation of the use of the Clarion multistrategy cochlear implant with the Hi-Focus electrode with positioner in adults and children. Sylmar: CA.

Bertram, B. 1996. Rehabilitation of children with cochlear implants with other disabilities. Presented at the International Symposium of Children with Cochlear implants. Hanover, Germany.

Bilger, R. C. Black, F. O. Hopkinson, N. T. Myers, E. N. Paynes, J. L., Stenson, N. R., Vega, A., and Wolf, R. V. 1977. Evaluation of subjects presently fitted with implanted auditory prostheses. *Annals of Otology, Rhinology and Laryngology* 86:3–10.

Bollard, P. M., Chute, P. M., Popp, A. L., and Parisier, S. C. 1999. Specific language growth in young children using the CLARION cochlear implant. *Annals of Otology, Rhinology and Laryngology* 177:119–23.

Chute, P. M. 2000. Cochlear implants in children with multiple handicapping conditions. Presented at the International Congress of Educators of the Deaf. Sydney, AU.

Chute, P. M., and Nevins, M. E. 1995. Cochlear implants in people who are deaf/blind. *Journal of Visually Impaired and Blind* 89:298–301.

Cochlear Corporation. 1999. *Package insert Nucleus 24 Cochlear Implant System.* Englewood, CO.

Cochlear Corporation. 2000. Investigational Device Exemption G990110. The Nucleus 24 contour adults and pediatric clinical trial. Englewood, CO.

Cowan, R. S. C., DelDot, J., Barker, E. J. et al. 1995. Speech perception in children using the advanced SPEAK speech-processing strategy. *Annals of Otology, Rhinology and Larynogology* 104:318–21.

Djourno, A., and Eyries, C. 1957. Prosthese auditive par excitation electrique a sistance du nerf sensoriel a L'aide d'un bobinage inclus a demeure. *Presse Med* 35:14–17.

Gantz, B. 2000. Early results of bilateral implantation in adults. Presented at the CI 2000 conference. Miami, FL.

Gantz, B. J., Tyler, R. S., Woodworth, G., Tye-Murray, N., and Fryauf-Bertschy, H. 1994. Results of multichannel cochlear implant in congenital and acquired prelingual deafness in children: Five year follow-up. *American Journal of Otology* 15:1–8.

Hodges, A. V., Schloffman, J., and Balkany, T. 1997. Conservation of residual hearing with cochlear implants. *American Journal of Otology* 18:179–83.

Kirk, K. I., Pisoni, D. B., and Osberger, M. J. 1995. Lexical effects on spoken word recognition by pediatric cochlear implant users. *Ear and Hearing* 16:470–81.

Lenarz, T. 1998. Cochlear implant selection criteria and shifting borders. *Acta Otorhinolaryngology* 52:83–199.

Mecklenburg, D., and Lehnhardt, E. 1996. Cochlear implant development in Europe, Asia, and Australia. In Cochlear Implants: A Practical Guide, ed. H. Cooper. San Diego: Singular Publishing Group.

Nevins, M. E., and Chute, P. C. 1996. Children with cochlear implants in educational settings. San Diego: Singular Publishing Group.

Niparko, J. 2000. Introduction. In *Cochlear Implants: Principles and Practice,* ed. J. Niparko. Philadelphia: Lippincott, Williams, and Wilkins.

Niparko, J., Cheng, A. K., and Francis, H. W. 2000. Outcomes of cochlear implantation: Assessment of quality of life impact and economic evaluation of the benefits of the cochlea implant in relation to costs. In *Cochlear Implants: Principles and Practice,* ed. J. Niparko. Philadelphia: Lippincott, Williams, and Wilkins.

National Institutes of Health Consensus Conference. Cochlear Implants 1995. *Journal of the American Medical Association* 274:1955–61.

Osberger, M. J., and Fisher, L. M. 1998. Preoperative predictors of postoperative implant performance in children. Presented at the 7th Symposium on Cochlear Implants in Children. Iowa City, IA.

Robbins, A. M. 1999. Language development. In *Cochlear implants,* eds. S. Waltzman and N. Cohen. New York: Thieme.

Sauberman, H. 2000. Food and Drug Administration approval process for cochlear implants. In *Cochlear Implants: Principles and Practice,* eds. J. Niparko et al. Philadelphia: Lippincott, Williams, and Wilkins.

Schindler, R. A., Kessler, K. D., Barker, M. 1995. Clarion patient performance: An update on the clinical trials. *Annals of Otology, Rhinology and Larngology* 166:269–72.

Staller, S. J., Menapace, C., Domico, E., et al. 1997. Speech perception abilities of adult and pediatric Nucleus implant recipients using Spectral Peak (SPEAK) coding strategy. *Otolaryngology, Head and Neck Surgery* 117:236–42.

Wilson, B. 2000. Strategies for representing speech information with cochlear implants. In *Cochlear Implants: Principles and Practice,* eds. J. Niparko et al. Philadelphia: Lippincott, Williams, and Wilkins.

Chapter ▪ 8

Intervention and Outcomes for Young Children Who Are Deaf and Hard of Hearing and Their Families

Mary Pat Moeller

We are entering a particularly optimistic era for the provision of early intervention services. There are technological advances resulting in much earlier identification of childhood hearing loss, improved amplification devices providing enhanced audibility, and increased opportunities for families to receive interventions that are responsive to family-identified needs. I will be exploring ways we might capitalize on this momentum to provide proactive, relationship-focused interventions for as many infants and families as possible. I will address early intervention issues from two perspectives, first, from a research perspective, what do we know about early intervention outcomes of the recent past, and what does this tell us about early intervention practice needs and, secondly, from a practical perspective. In this section, I will explore some struggles and strategies we have identified in our efforts to become increasingly family-centered with the majority of families.

But, as I look ahead to the potentially bright future for infants and families, I am reminded of some lessons that we must remember, even when early intervention models come wrapped in shiny new packages. I mention these timeless lessons because we are honoring Dr. David Luterman, who taught us so many of these lessons. His visionary leadership in working with families has spread like ripples in a pool to touch countless lives. The lessons I learned from David Luterman stick with me—they goad me, in fact, when I catch myself making old, familiar mistakes with families. I want to highlight just a few of these elegant and timeless lessons because they speak so well to current issues in intervention.

Timeless lesson number one: Luterman often says, "If families do well, children will do well." Family focused from the start, long before the term "family centered" came in vogue, he appreciates that children live in a family system and that transactions surrounding a child's disability affect the system as a whole. So he focuses on families first, and knows that if families fare well, so will kids. He provides the psycho-social support that allows families to adapt to their circumstances and get on with living. He long ago set the model for encouraging families to explore all their options and he reminds us that "parents are smart and they will choose wisely." He has known for a long time that decision-making authority rests with the family.

Timeless lesson number two: Once I was giving a presentation about the multi-disciplinary team process we had implemented at Boys Town for evaluating deaf and hard-of-hearing children, and David Luterman was in the audience. I remember his gentle guidance to this day (and this is timeless lesson number two): "It's only the families with the greatest ego strength that can withstand a multi-disciplinary team process." Dr. Don Bailey, a noted expert on early intervention and family-centered practices, shared his own feelings of intimidation when attending educational planning meetings for his special needs daughter (Bailey 1995). We should remember this lesson and consider how to meet individual needs.

Timeless lesson number three: Some members of our staff were expressing concern about the fact that only the parents who did not really need it were showing up for our family sign class. Then I remembered David Luterman's words, "If you create a program that really meets family's needs, they will come." He developed programs in response to family-identified needs. Once we stopped designing programs based on what we thought parents needed, the impact increased greatly. As an example, through listening to parents, we made our way past the traditional parent sign class to create a multi-faceted approach to supporting families with sign instruction. Families are able to choose the approaches that best meet their needs. The offerings range from class nights (with the grandparent and sibling/neighborhood classes being among the most popular), Deaf mentors working with families on storytelling strategies, videotaped materials, and family weekends. Lesson formats focus on placing conversational interaction tools in the hands of families, not on lists of vocabulary. David Luterman was right—if you build it, they will come. He knew that it needed to be built in a variety of forms.

Timeless lesson number four: This one has brought comic relief to many a beleaguered parent of a toddler. I can hear David Luterman saying, "You know there's nothing deafer than a typical two-year-old." He has shown us many ways to support families in their efforts to put deafness in perspective within the family. I find it instructive to consider how visionary these lessons are. They give us insights into the "hows" of family-centered practice.

With these lessons in mind, I first turn to some recent research on early intervention outcomes and their implications for early intervention practice.

EARLY INTERVENTION OUTCOMES

Variables affecting Child Outcomes

A primary goal of early intervention is to make use of sensitive periods of development in infancy in order to prevent the language, academic, and social delays that often accompany late-identified sensorineural hearing loss (Blair, Peterson, and Viehweg 1985; Davis et al. 1986; Leavitt and McGarr 1988; Moeller et al. 1981; Moeller et al. 1996). Yoshinaga-Itano and her colleagues (1998) demonstrated that many children with sensorineural hearing loss are able to achieve language abilities similar to hearing peers if they have access to quality intervention services prior to six months of age. There is increasing and widespread support for the notion that children with hearing loss benefit from proactive management, beginning with universal newborn hearing screening (NIH 1993; Joint Committee on Infant Hearing 1994; American Academy of Pediatrics 1999).

Arguments over the sensibility of proceeding with universal newborn hearing screening focused on the fact that there was limited empirical evidence that early intervention (EI) makes a lasting difference for children and families (Bess and Paradise 1994). This provoked a resurgence of interest in determining if EI makes meaningful differences in the lives of families, and also in identifying variables that contribute to positive outcomes. Gurlanick (1997) pointed out that many critical questions related to principles and practices of early intervention remained unanswered or completely unexplored. He stresses the need for a new generation of research that examines the influence of program features, and of child and family characteristics, on the specific outcomes and goals of early intervention. In other words, how do specific aspects of intervention interact with individual child and family factors to bring about positive outcomes? We use this general term "early intervention," yet it is unreasonable to assume that all interventions are created equal and that they are all one and the same (Carney 1996). What is it about various intervention approaches that work, and for whom do they work? Calderon and Greenberg (1997) have suggested that elements of programs rarely studied, such as process-type factors that are consistent across successful programs, might make the greatest difference. An example of a "process type" factor may be the quality of the relationship developed between the family and the early intervention personnel. Calderon and Greenberg note that an especially important factor may be the ability of an early interventionist to have an impact on the parents' sense of self efficacy in relating to the deaf child and professionals; to influence parents' sense of hopefulness about the situation; and to foster realistic and positive expectations. As we enter this era where more children enter the system early, these multidimensional issues of outcome deserve our attention.

Now let us look at some recent research findings and what they reveal about child outcomes, family outcomes, and parent-professional partnerships in intervention. First, I will review selected results of a retrospective analysis of early intervention outcomes from children who are graduates of our program (Moeller 2000).[1] Three questions were asked:

1. Is there a relationship between age of enrollment in intervention and language outcomes at age five? If so, do the earliest identified children maintain a language advantage through age five?
2. What variables, in addition to early intervention, influence outcomes?
3. Is there a relationship between family involvement and language outcomes?

One hundred and twelve children (58 males, 54 females) who were graduates of the Diagnostic Early Intervention Program in Omaha, Nebraska were included in the study. This group of children did not have the benefit of universal newborn hearing screening, and the average age of identification was 1.55 years (approximately 18 months). The average age of entry was 1.83 years or approximately 22 months (range .03—4.53 years). All of the children had congenital, bilateral sensorineural hearing loss that ranged from mild to profound. The distribution by degree of hearing loss is unlike the expected distribution in that 47 of 112 children had profound degrees of hearing loss and only 9 had mild hearing loss. This distributional spread is in

[1]This previously published work is summarized with permission from *Pediatrics*.

part a result of limited availability of services for children with profound hearing loss in sparsely populated areas of the state, prompting parents to relocate to areas where comprehensive services are provided. It may also reflect the inconsistent provision of specialized services for children with mild degrees of hearing loss.

In this study, 63 of the families had chosen to enroll their children in an auditory-oral program; 51 families selected a signing program. These two community-based programs implemented parallel curricular approaches from birth through five years of age.

We were interested in determining the status of the children's vocabulary and verbal reasoning skills upon entry to kindergarten, because we know that these skills are particularly relevant to literacy development (Davis 1942). Dependent measures included a receptive vocabulary measure, the Peabody Picture Vocabulary Test, (PPVT, Dunn 1981) and the Preschool Language Assessment Instrument (PLAI, Blank, Rose, and Berlin 1978), which had been administered to a representative subset of 80 of the participants. These measures correlated well with the children's scores on an expressive vocabulary measure, ($r = .81$, $p < .01$), and with performance on global measures of receptive and expressive language (either the Reynell Developmental Language Scales [Reynell 1977] or the Preschool Language Scale [Zimmerman, Steiner, and Pond 1992]), ($r = .80$, $p < .01$). In addition, for 92% of the participants, the PPVT was the lowest of the set of scores, making this a conservative estimate.

The verbal reasoning test (PLAI) that was used examines children's abilities to respond to discourse demands that commonly occur in kindergarten classrooms. Test items range from simple to abstract in terms of their cognitive-linguistic complexity. For example, at the basic level, a child sees a picture of a pair of scissors and is asked to label it ("What is this?"). At the next level, the child is asked a question like, "What do you do with this?" For level three, the examiner points to the screw on the scissors and asks, "What do you think this part is for?" Level four is the most abstract level and became the primary focus of this investigation. To illustrate, the child is presented with a picture (e.g., a child pouring juice into a bottomless cup accompanied by five geometric shapes, one solid, some odd shapes or with holes). The child is then asked to reason in response to a question like, "Which of these things could we use to fix the cup? Why did you pick that one?" This fourth level requires that the child not only understand an abstract question, but be able to formulate a reason to justify his or her answer. This highest level of reasoning was the focus of the current study.

A rating scale was developed in an attempt to characterize the level and quality of family involvement in the program. Many of us have witnessed the contributions families make to their children's progress. Intuitively it made sense that this variable may be contributing to outcome along with other variables of interest. Each family received a global rating of 1 to 5 to reflect their participation in the early intervention program. Ratings were assigned independently by two early interventionists who had extensive contact with the family for a period of two years and often as much as four years. Judges were given specific descriptions of characteristics representing each category prior to assigning ratings (Moeller 2000). A rating of 5, for example, was assigned when involvement was "ideal." Such families demonstrated active and independent engagement in sessions. They were highly effective communication partners with their infants, sought out information, had support from extended "family," and in general demonstrated evidence of positive adjustment. A family rated 3, or "average," had basic facility in conversing with the child, needed continued support in using language facilitation techniques, and demonstrated limited carryover of principles due to other stressors. Family involvement characterized on the lowest end of the scale applied to situations where the family faced significant life stressors that took precedence over the child's communicative needs (e.g., domestic violence, homelessness). In general, at this end of the scale, understanding of the child's deafness was limited, participation in sessions was sporadic, and communication was limited to only the most basic needs. Cohen's Kappa was calculated to examine inter-judge reliability for the family ratings. Levels of agreement were 88% and 94% for the oral and signing programs, respectively.

The main findings are summarized in relation to the original questions. First of all, is there a relationship between age of enrollment and language outcomes at age five? The answer is yes for both vocabulary and verbal reasoning performance. A significant negative correlation ($r = -.46, p < .01$) was found between age of enrollment and vocabulary. Later enrollment was associated with lower levels of performance at age five, irrespective of the degree of hearing loss. A significant negative correlation was also found between verbal reasoning skills and age of enrollment ($r = -.31, p < .01$).

Furthermore, the findings support the results of Yoshinaga-Itano et al. (1998) in that the earliest enrolled children (defined in this study as < 12 months) obtained vocabulary scores that were within the average range compared to hearing peers (Mean Standard Score = 93.6). There was an effect size for vocabulary of one standard deviation when the early group was compared to children enrolled between 2 and 3 years, and 1.6 standard deviations for children identified after 3 years. These effect sizes are also similar to those reported by Yoshinaga-Itano et al. (1998). This suggests an affirmative answer to the second part of the question. Differences between the early- and later-identified groups maintained themselves through age five. However, there is a difficult-to-control confound in studies that compare children identified early and later. The children identified later have less time in intervention. This must be kept in mind when interpreting results. Arguably, late identification may leave us in a situation of having insufficient time for children to establish linguistic readiness for literacy by the time they enter school.

Notably, the results of this study showed a systematic decline in the mean vocabulary standard scores with increasing ages of enrollment, as illustrated in figure 1. Similar results were found for the verbal reasoning measure. Earliest identified children scored within the low average range (25th percentile) compared to hearing five-year olds on abstract reasoning, and there was a systematic decline in performance with increasing ages of enrollment. The fact that the children scored in the low average range on verbal reasoning leads to cautious interpretations of statements that the children "performed like hearing peers." These results point to some important qualitative differences in the language abilities of these two groups of children. It is also clear from figure 1 that there is considerable variability in individual performance along the age of enrollment continuum. This observation led us to consider what variables, in addition to age of enrollment, may be contributing to variance.

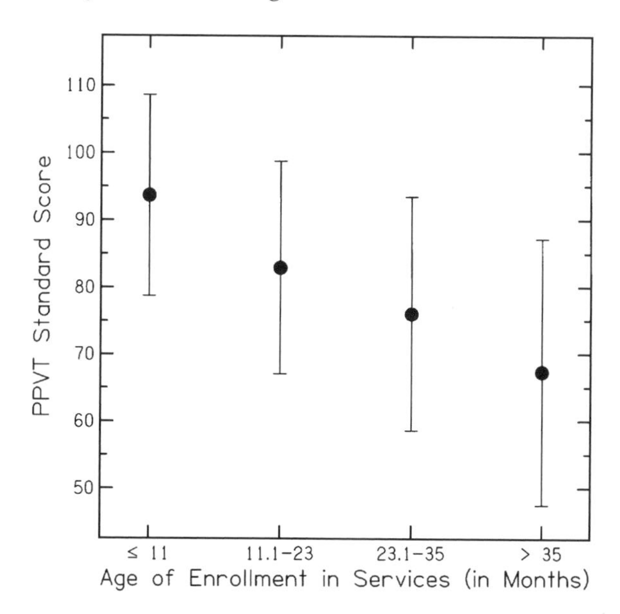

Figure 1. Means and standard deviations of PPVT scores for subjects as a function of age of enrollment in intervention. Reprinted with permission from *Pediatrics*.

Multiple regression models were applied to explore the collective and separate effects of various background factors on children's language outcomes at age five. The four variables of age of enrollment, family involvement, better ear pure tone average, and nonverbal intelligence explained 55% of the variance in vocabulary scores. However, only two of the targeted variables contributed significantly to explained variance: age of enrollment (R^2 change = .114, $p < .001$) and family involvement (R^2 change = .352, $p < .001$). The family involvement variable was the strongest contributor. This explained why some children who were identified later showed a pattern of "catching up." They tended to be from the families with highest involvement. Notably, the opposite was also true; some early-identified children who made slow gains were from families with lower levels of involvement.

Importantly, there is an interaction between the variables of age of enrollment and family involvement that influences outcomes. Figure 2 shows vocabulary standard scores as a function of both contributing variables. The earliest-enrolled children performed better

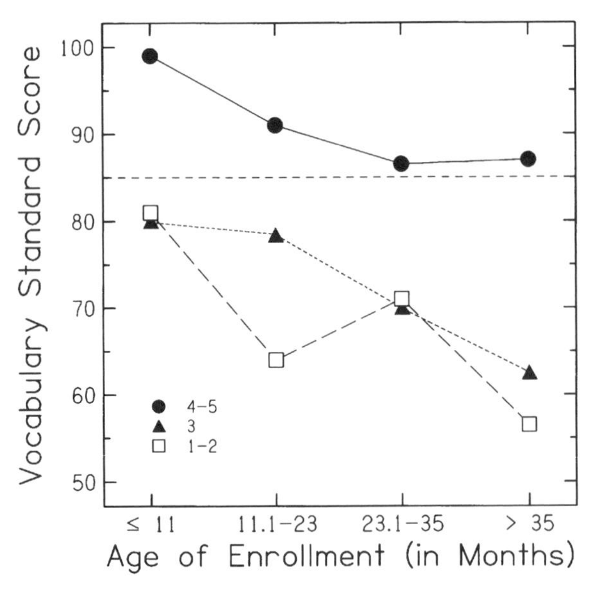

Figure 2. Mean vocabulary scores plotted as a function of the two key variables, age of enrollment and family involvement ratings. The area above the horizontal dashed line represents the lower end of the average range for normal hearing students (average range is 100 ± 15). 4–5 (filled circle) represents highest levels of family involvement; 3 (filled triangle) represents average family involvement; 1–2 (open square) represents below average family involvement. Reprinted with permission from *Pediatrics*.

than later-enrolled children across all levels of family involvement, underscoring the importance of early enrollment. However, it is encouraging to see that strong family involvement had a kind of buffering effect when enrollment was late. Although getting into services late is not optimal, these families appeared to make up for lost time. This finding may give encouragement to families who, despite universal hearing screenings, access services later. With that said, however, I raise the question of the cost to the family of a child identified later in terms of stress, guilt, frustrations of not being listened to, and pressures to "catch up." There is also evidence that many families experience behavioral difficulties with their children when identification is late and communication is delayed (Mertens, Sass-Lehrer, and Scott-Olson 2000). Late identification is costly not just in terms of child outcome, but also family outcome.

These data suggest that children identified later, from families rated average or below for involvement, are at particular risk. The mean standard scores of these two groups fell between 56.5 and 62, or more than two standard deviations behind their peers at kindergarten entry. Optimum outcomes were observed when children had the combined advantages of early enrollment and strong family involvement. The results support the need for early identification programs that are paired with interventions that seek to involve families.

It is possible that the effects of age of enrollment may be even greater when groups who have the advantage of universal newborn hearing screenings (UNHS) are followed longitudinally, as the Colorado group is doing. The retrospective analysis I am discussing included only 24 children in the earliest-identified group.[2]

It also must be kept in mind that the results of this study and those of Yoshinaga-Itano et al. (1998) were obtained in response to comprehensive interventions, typically provided by experienced professionals. In the case of the Omaha study, families received home-bound intervention services 1 to 2 times per week, had access to a parent support group, and for signing families, there was a weekly family sign program. The role that comprehensive interventions play in outcomes needs further investigation. It cannot be assumed that early identification alone will bring about desired outcomes.

[2]At Boys Town National Research Hospital (BTNRH) we have recently initiated a longitudinal prospective study of children with mild to moderately severe hearing loss (HH) compared to a control group of hearing infants. These efforts should avoid some of the problems inherent in retrospective analyses (such as comparing children who have different levels of intervention) and should address some of the unanswered questions about children with milder degrees of loss.

Some additional analyses of these data lend support to this conclusion. I was interested in looking at whether children in the program were closing the gap between language age and chronological age following intervention. To examine this, I looked at receptive and expressive language measures (Reynell Development Language Scale or Preschool Language Scale) administered annually between the ages of 2 and 5. Following the lead of Yoshinaga-Itano et al. (1998), I calculated language quotients as a measure of the extent of language delay. Receptive language quotients were derived by dividing language age by chronological age and multiplying by 100. If the child obtains a receptive language quotient (LQ) of 100, then chronological age and language age are equal (the score is age appropriate). If a child obtains a language quotient of 80, then language age is delayed in comparison to chronological age. At five years of age, a LQ of 80 would translate to an age equivalent of 4 years or approximately one year delayed. Figure 3 contains average receptive language quotients across time with the children grouped by age of enrollment in the program. It illustrates that, on average, the children in the study showed a pattern over time of closing the gap between chronological age and language age. However, the gains are more pronounced and result in age-appropriate functioning only for the children in the earliest enrolled group. The same trends were observed for expressive language. Note that there were some strong performers in the 24 to 35 month group,

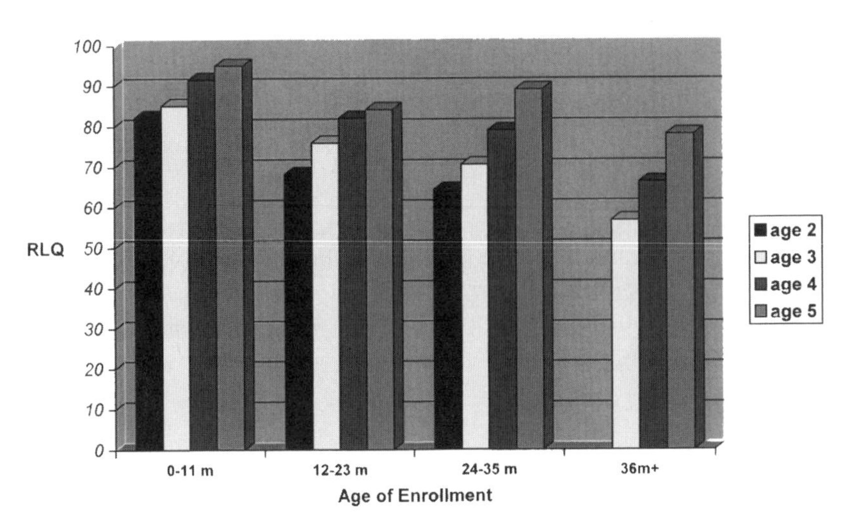

Figure 3. Average receptive language quotients for the children at ages 2, 3, 4 and 5, clustered by ages of enrollment in the program.

which shows a somewhat stronger growth pattern than the 12 to 23 month group. This was influenced by individual subjects in this group with strong family involvement and lesser degrees of hearing loss. Figure 4 shows the same data plotted by age at test date. This again demonstrates the advantage for the children identified early.

I was also interested in looking at the characteristics of children who scored at various levels on verbal reasoning skills. The 80 subjects who received this test were divided into three nearly equal groups by those scoring at or above the 25th percentile (*N* = 27), between the 10 and 25th percentiles (*N* = 27), and at or below the 1st percentile (*N* = 26). Table I compares these subject groups on the background variables of interest. These results suggest that earlier identifications and family involvement play a particularly important role in the development of verbal reasoning skills.

The data present a fairly cohesive picture of the importance of the two original variables identified, that of early enrollment and family involvement, as contributors to outcome. They suggest that early intervention makes a difference for the majority of children, and they support the need for early interventions to focus on the involvement of families in ways that enhance communicative interactions. This conclusion is

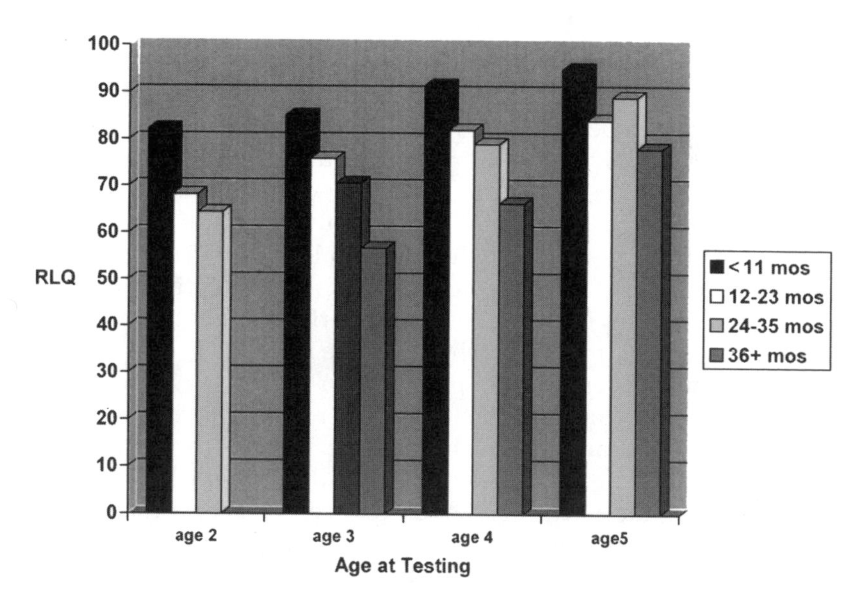

Figure 4. Comparison of the receptive language quotients of children from various age-of-enrollment categories on their performance at ages 2, 3, 4 and 5 years.

Table I. Characteristics of children scoring at various levels on a test of verbal reasoning (mean scores are represented in the table).

Performance Category	Age of Enrollment	Family Involvement Rating	Better Ear Pure Tone Average
Highest performers (At or above 25th%ile)	1.2 years	4.4 years	71 dB
Average perfomers (10th to 25th %ile)	1.8 years	3.6	75 dB
Low performers	2.3 years	2.6	80 dB

supported by the recent findings of Calderon (2000). She examined the relationship between family involvement in deaf and hard of hearing children's school programs and child outcomes in language and academics. This was an analysis of 28 families who graduated from the same early intervention program. She found that family involvement in school functions like IEP meetings predicted child outcomes. But more importantly, maternal communication skills were the strongest predictor of language and academic functioning. Calderon concluded that professionals should seek to involve families in programs with the goal of enhancing parental communication skills with the child.

Variable affecting Family Outcomes

We need to know much more about the impact of intervention on families. Calderon, Bargones, and Sidman (1998) completed further analysis of 28 families who graduated from the same early intervention program. They used multiple procedures, including child language assessments, parent and teacher questionnaires, parent interviews, record reviews, and videotaped analysis of parent-child interaction. The authors concluded that families involved in early intervention represent a highly heterogenous group, fitting no single profile. The strong implication is that early intervention must be viewed as a flexible tool that is shaped to the individual family profile.

Their subjects entered the program, on average, at 21 months of age. An issue they raised is that families entering this late receive a limited amount of early intervention service. Families from rural areas were particularly at risk to receive reduced services when entering late. Assuming the early intervention services are successful in shaping effective communicative interactions in families, what are the consequences for families accessing services for perhaps one-third of the intended birth-to-three-year period? These authors found that many of the families in their study were only moderately involved with the early intervention objectives. They were able to follow the interventionists' lead but did not demonstrate high levels of confidence or independence in enhancing the child's skills. This study raises a number of practical questions. What type and intensity of service fosters parental independence in nurturing the child's communication? Given a highly diverse population, how do interventionists find the best fit of approaches for families? What is the impact of late identification on the dynamics of parent/infant interaction? We need a better understanding of the issues of timing and intensity of early intervention in relation to outcomes for families.

Another recent report points to the positive impact fathers have on outcomes for children. Calderon and Low (1998) looked specifically at the fathers' involvement in 22 families and found that the presence of a father in the home facilitated deaf children's academic and language outcomes. Previous studies have suggested that fathers influence children only indirectly by providing additional support to the mother (Schilling et al. 1986). However, Calderon and Low (1998) found that fathers may have a direct influence on their children's communicative development, even though fathers in this study rated themselves as less proficient in signing skills than the mothers. It was concluded that the daily father-child interactions involved in trying to establish shared communication are sufficient to be of benefit to the child. The implication is that involvement of fathers should be an integral goal of early intervention, and it may take nontraditional approaches to better address this issue. We will discuss this a bit further when considering practical intervention strategies.

Parental-Professional Partnerships—What do we know?

Qualitative methods were implemented to examine mothers' expectations of early intervention and interventionists (Dromi and Ingber 1999). Fifty Israeli mothers of young deaf children who had been enrolled in family centered early-intervention programs for at least one year participated in this study. Research techniques included open-ended written questions, a follow-up personal interview, and a demographic questionnaire. They found that mothers expressed a wide range of expectations of programs and professionals. A particularly unique aspect of the analysis was the application of cluster analysis to classify mothers into four distinctive groups based on shared expectations. The first group was described as *Independent Decision Makers* (N = 7). This group of mothers demonstrated high confidence in their abilities and the desire to take full responsibility for decisions. They viewed professionals as useful resources to be exploited, and viewed themselves as carrying the primary responsibility for the child's intervention and wanted to be fully involved in decision making. A second group was characterized as *Well Socialized* (*N* = 13). These mothers were described as fully accepting of and satisfied with their current intervention program. They wanted some level of involvement in the child's intervention, but their desire for partnership with professionals was not as developed as other groups. A third group (*N* = 23) included mothers who seemed to want to relinquish responsibility for the intervention. They were observed to be passive and had less tendency to become involved in intervention. Instead of asking for control or involvement, they saw the professional as fully responsible for the planning and implementing the intervention. These mothers did not expect counseling for themselves. They viewed the child as the client. A final group (*N* = 7) was classified as *Full Collaborators* who seemed to understand the complexity of the intervention process and the value of collaboration with professionals. They attributed the decision-making role to the professional, but wanted significant input and respect for their input. They held an attitude of openness to learning from professionals and were interested in receiving psychosocial support. In general, mothers wanted information, guidance, and support, and expected that professionals would be well-trained and strong in interpersonal support skills. The four subgroups differed, then, with respect to who should be the target of early intervention. The results suggest that families may come to intervention with different expectations from the professional about roles, about who is the client, and about how they will interact with the early interventionist (Dromi and Ingber 1999). Professionals and families may encounter value conflicts over what is important in the intervention process (Bailey 1987; Mertens, Sass-Lehrer, and Scott-Olson 2000).

It is not known if the experiences of Israeli mothers can be generalized to mothers in the United States; however, that we must clarify parents' expectations of professionals certainly can be generalized. To what degree are these outcomes a result of individual differences in style, coping, and experience? How might the intervention experience itself influence perceptions? Are there ways to influence perceptions in order to encourage the active involvement of families?

Family-centered programs seek to involve families directly in intervention. Yet, EI programs vary in the extent of focus on parental involvement. McBride and Peterson (1997) observed the home visit strategies of 15 early interventionists serving 18 families with special needs children (non-deaf/hard of hearing). Observations of 160 sessions indicated that early interventionists primarily worked directly with children, although often in conjunction with a parent. The researchers concluded that a child-focused model of early intervention was being implemented. They added that the interventionists were functioning as the key change agent and there was little, if any, emphasis on support of the parent-child relationship. These findings are of concern if we recognize that the impact of early intervention may not be at its optimum when implemented with the family as a "spectator sport."

In another study of early intervention outcomes in special education, four early intervention programs were evaluated in relation to their impact on parent-child interaction (Mahoney et al. 1998). Results indicated that the impact of interventions on children's development was directly related to their effectiveness at *supporting* and *encouraging* parents to engage in responsive interactions with their child. They found that maternal responsiveness to the child was consistently associated with significant child outcomes. Interestingly, their findings provided little support for child-focused, directive teaching models. The researchers maintained that there is widespread reluctance on the part of early intervention professionals to incorporate relationship-focused concepts into practice (Mahoney et al. 1998).

We may find good agreement among this audience that a primary goal of early intervention should be to promote sensitive and responsive transactions between infants and family members. We have historical evidence showing that interactions between hearing mothers and deaf children can be problematic. Hearing mothers have been characterized in the literature as being directive and controlling (see Gallaway and Woll 1994, for a review). More recent research has challenged this notion, demonstrating that this behavior is an intuitive adaptation mothers make to the deaf child's language delay. In fact, hearing mothers of deaf children used response controls (e.g., commands) to the same level as mothers of language-matched hearing children (Cross, Nienhuys, and Kirkman 1985).

Lederberg and Prezbindowski (2000) point out that negative characterizations of hearing mothers in the literature may bias early interventionists toward focusing on negative aspects of interactions. They recommend identification of intuitive parenting strengths in the family (Koester and Papousek 2000) and use of a balanced approach that fosters parents' natural competencies to communicate while identifying some areas of need. There is evidence that hearing mothers do make some natural adaptations to their child's communicative needs (Spencer and Lederberg 1998), yet these adaptations may not be sufficient for optimal communication (Koester and Papousek 2000). Deaf parents are often skilled at adapting to the visual communication needs of their deaf infants (Koester, Karkowski, and Traci 1998; Koester et al. 2000). This has led early intervention programs using sign language to form partnerships with deaf mentors, who guide hearing families in the use of strategies for attention getting, negotiation of joint attention, and increasing visual accessibility for deaf babies (Mohay 2000). There is evidence that this approach results in improved outcomes for children as well (Watkins, Pittman, and Walden 1998).

Collectively, these findings underscore the importance of relationship-focused interventions where families' strengths are identified and supported to foster responsive transactions. The value of careful observation of what is already going well between parents and children is underscored. I recall my early parent-infant days when I arrived at a home with a carefully planned agenda to teach the parent how to interact. I never stopped long enough to recognize what was already going well. Later I made the important discovery that observing and pointing out parents' intuitive skills built their confidence in interacting with the child. Although there is much to be learned, the literature provides theoretical support for many of the key principles of family-centered practice.

EARLY INTERVENTION AS A PROCESS

Family-centered early intervention starts with relationship building. The next sections explore premises underlying this process and practical strategies for implementing the approach. These techniques are based on the collaborative efforts of Moeller and Condon (1994, 1998).

Premise One: Family-Centered Practice is a process. It evolves in unique ways with each family through time, commitment, and willingness to adapt. At the inception of the Diagnostic Early Intervention Project (DEIP) at Boys Town National Research Hospital, we wanted to build a community-based team that would provide support to families in coping with the diagnosis and in gathering information to empower family decision making. Families enroll for a period of at least 6 months in what we try to shape as a kind of "comfort zone." Families are given time and support to gather information, to gain a better understanding of the child's needs in relation to family needs, and to use the team as a sounding board as they explore possibilities. This team started with some solid ideas, but the emergence of family-centered practice concepts has challenged us to evolve to a new level in working with families. Like other teams, we had to recognize child-focused aspects of our program model and move increasingly toward the spirit of family-centered care. I want to highlight a few practical strategies that continue to facilitate this process, in the hope that they might assist other teams in the process of transition. By team, I am referring to the transdisciplinary team (including parents, an audiologist, a speech-language pathologist, services coordinator, parent/infant educator, and local program administrators).

1. *It is invaluable to invest in training teams as teams.* It is particularly useful to ask teams to generalize established principles

of family-centered practice to their own situation. In some cases, attitudes have to be changed. Thinking about *how* these principles could work in our situation was critical. We had to recognize that we had a history of "calling the shots" so to speak—of *advising* parents about their children instead of learning how families wanted to proceed. We recognized the need to be more consumer driven and less professionally prescribed.

I clearly remember the day I recognized that we were evolving. It was the day a 16-year-old single mother described her seven-month old to other members of the team. The admiration she had for her little one came through loud and clear. It was followed by a direct description of what she wanted next. In effect, she was calling the shots and the team was highly motivated to support her. Not all families participate with our team in this manner, but it struck me that before this evolution, very few would even try.

2. *It is useful to recognize a team's strengths and draw on these to build interdependence.* As a specific example, our team has an excellent Services Coordinator. At first, her knowledge of deafness was limited, yet her capacity to learn from other team members is limitless. It might have been easy for us to take the position that she had little to offer because she was not an "expert" in deafness. And how wrong we would have been. Lessons we learn from her are among the most valuable: how to listen sensitively for family needs and priorities, and how to flex and bend our typical approaches to meet unique needs. She is one of the family's first contacts with the early intervention system and the comfort they feel in her presence at the team meetings is obvious. In our experience, Services Coordinators make vital contributions to the team's ability to address the needs of the family system as a whole.
3. *The team needs to devote time to meta-analysis.* We stop every few months and ask ourselves, "How are we doing as a team? Is there anything we need to change?" These discussions are aided by feedback recruited from families.
4. *It is important to recognize that it takes time for teams to develop the level of trust that results in successful conflict resolution and increasing interdependence.* Hall and Loucks (1978) described some steps that people often experience in accepting and investing in change. Awareness that there is a need for change is a first step in the process. Collaboration is a much later step, so it may be unrealistic to expect that early on. In order

to reach that level, team members benefit from gathering information, addressing personal concerns about the change, and identifying managerial solutions to possible pitfalls. It can also be useful to observe the consequences of the change in other successful programs, giving team members a joint vision for change. Collaboration is more likely once team members have this vision and are invested in the change and in working together. When our team members became invested in the goal of identifying and supporting family needs and decisions, it became easier to consider each other's viewpoints.

The next premises address the relationship that develops between the parent-infant specialist and the family. As Calderon and Greenberg (1997) pointed out, this may be a particularly critical variable in the success of early interventions. In this section, I will explore some specific relationship building techniques.

Premise Two: Relationships between family members and professionals should reflect partnerships. These may take different forms, but should have a foundation built on honesty, respect, trust, reciprocity, and open communication. Trainers from the Family Enablement Project (1991) described some minimal requirements of family-professional partnerships: (1) Both the family and the professional want to and agree to enter into a collaborative arrangement. Not all families will desire a partnership, but our challenge is to try to build toward partnerships whenever we can to benefit families. We may need to recognize common barriers to partnership that may exist in role perceptions and remove them; (2) Both families and professionals contribute resources and expertise, including knowledge, skill, and time; and (3) The process needs to be decided at the point of entry and the locus of control in decision making clearly stated. The logical conclusion is that much of this process relies on the relationship building skills of the interventionist who is attempting to be a partner with a diverse array of families. It also suggests that partners need to be clear at the outset and negotiate how the relationship might proceed. Personally, I find it useful to share with families my expectations for how we will come together in intervention, because it may represent quite a departure from what they are expecting. Considering parental expectations helps us find a common ground. Many parents come to professionals (e.g., a doctor) expecting them to take charge, diagnose, advise, and then back off. But here we are, wanting a relationship that builds parental confidence and we plan to hang around for the road ahead. This means we need to set a tone of shared expertise from the first visit, if we want a partnership to form. In other words, we want to balance the relationship to the degree possible to avoid a professional-as-expert relationship.

The first few visits are particularly critical in setting the tone for the subsequent relationship building. Initial contacts are typically devoted to becoming acquainted, establishing a caring atmosphere, conveying that parents' needs are heard by using focused, active listening, clarifying family's expectations and concerns, and discussing roles. Throughout early sessions, an important goal is to establish a quality relationship between parents and professional, while being sensitive to the fact that the parents are still reeling from the impact of identification (Moeller and Condon 1994).

I believe our goal is to create a situation with families and infants where both parties are comfortable implementing relationship-focused interventions. This is accomplished when parents spend time in the "driver's seat" during sessions (e.g., directly interacting with the baby) and the interventionist is watching, learning, and guiding. We find that some parents are more comfortable when the interventionist dives in and works directly with the child. Perhaps parents lack confidence and feel vulnerable when the clinician is watching them. We want to establish a comfortable way of working with each other from the start that conveys that we are sharing ideas and expertise, not judging or evaluating parenting skills.

When asked, many parent/infant educators will confirm that they find it easier to work directly with the child. But what is the down side of such an approach? In some cases, it can undermine parental sense of competence and control. It can foster dependency rather than independent skills. It may also shift the focus unnecessarily in initial contacts toward the child and specific content, instead of allowing parents to share feelings and be heard. It also puts us in the position of giving the "most help" right away, before we have observed, listened, and understood.

Relationship-building techniques

Some specific relationship building skills can be used by the interventionist to get partnerships started, such as *structuring the context to allow for non-intrusive gathering of information*. During early visits, we find it helpful to set up a natural play situation where the clinician is on the sidelines and has a chance to learn from the parents as they engage the baby in typical routines. The clinician follows the lead of parent and child and uses focused attention techniques. Conversation is directed toward parental statements and infant behavior, rather than new information or the experiences of others. During such sessions, the clinician brings diagnostic expertise to the mix. While observing, it is particularly valuable for the clinician to watch and listen for: (1) cultural and family values; (2) names of supportive people; (3) coping strategies the family uses; (4) what the family wants us to do next; (5) ways that the family has solved problems in the past; (6) evaluation questions on the parents' minds; (7) strengths of the family in adjusting to the child's diagnosis; and (8) strengths of the family in caring for the child and meeting his or her needs (Condon 1997). These observations aid the clinician in building toward an IFSP.

A second technique involves *actively recruiting and accepting parents' perceptions, interpretations, and advice about the infant, even when the perception differs from that of the clinician.* This technique is especially helpful in conveying an attitude that sharing of expertise is desired. In one example, a clinician observed a toddler responding to the sound of a toy. At the same time, the mother reported, "He didn't hear it."[3] The clinician responded by inviting the mother to elaborate ("you don't think so?). The mother answered, "No, because if he did he would be interested in how it came out." Notice that the clinician invited more input by asking an open-ended question. This technique allows the clinician to discover how the mother is thinking about her toddler's hearing responses and what evidence she values. This input will contribute insight when they explore the limits of his hearing responses and work to build consensus. It is also useful to recruit parental concerns through open-ended questioning. I remember one of the families I worked with waited until five minutes before the end of each session to bring up a number of important affective concerns. I learned to start sessions with open-ended questions like, "What have you been thinking about since our last visit," or "Has anything been on your mind that we can talk about?" This conveyed the idea that the infant was not our sole purpose for coming together, and that my role is to provide family support.

Another valuable relationship-building skill is to *provide objective feedback about the interaction.* This also helps to build an atmosphere of mutual respect for skills and knowledge. Importantly, the feedback avoids judgmental comments, and instead gives a description of what is happening. For example, the clinician states, "I notice that you use his word back to him so he knows he was understood. I've seen him smile several times when you do that. I bet that feels really good to him." This type of feedback is often reinforcing to the parent and can bolster confidence that their intuitive parenting is on the right track. These skills may be so automatic that they are not consciously recognized as a strength. This sharing of objective feedback also lets the parent know that the clinician is a skilled, credible observer. This can

[3]Quotes are taken from a training videotape produced by Condon and Moeller (unpublished).

support the goal of striving for mutuality in making suggestions or observations. It can also be useful to summarize observations near the end of a session as a goal-focusing strategy. Some interventionists come up with a brief written summary entitled, "things we have worked on together today." This can serve as a helpful record and reminder of key points, but it can also reinforce the notion of shared expertise and partnership.

When either partner identifies a diagnostic question, a powerful tool can be the *use of joint discovery through experiments.* Through joint experiments, partners have a tool for discovering what does or does not work with the infant (Schuyler and Rushmer 1987). It also serves as a non-directive way to guide the parent-infant interaction and avoid the feeling of evaluation. For example, the interventionist observes that offering the child an alternative might calm his behavior. There are three choices in this situation: The interventionist can offer the child the alternate toy and succeed in calming him, although, this comes with the risk of missing opportunities to see if the suggestion will work for the parent; a second choice is to tell the parent what to do especially early-on, this can give an impression of professional-as-expert. A final strategy is to respectfully pose the strategy as a question that can be explored through experimentation. "I wonder what will happen if you offer him an alternative? I wonder if he might calm down?" This invites the parent to try a skill and gives both partners feedback on its effectiveness. It is particularly valuable when the parents adopt the same process as their own way to discover what works. For example, a mother informed and showed the clinician that her son was not likely to respond to visual stimulation on the right side of his head. Earlier in the session, no concern for vision had been expressed in response to questions. Her statement of concern about vision came about in the natural process of experimenting. The clinician followed up the observation with an invitation for elaboration. "Now will you show me how he responds on the left side?" and added upon watching the result, "You certainly are observant." By inviting this final "experiment" the clinician again conveyed respect for the mother's expertise.

Experiments can also be initiated as a way to resolve a conflict or test out decisions. Sometimes parents have ideas and desires that conflict with the way we see things. By setting up a mini experiment, we can see how the child responds to the suggested approach. Experiments lead to observations that inform rather than to content-focused tussles over whose view is right or wrong. Suppose that the parent of an infant persists in making requests for child-focused speech intervention as part of the IFSP. The professional believes that this will be developmentally inappropriate. It may be that the parent is feeling particularly anxious about the child's progress. Speech therapy may be viewed as a way to "fix" an observable concern. It will be important to explore parental expectations and fears. It may also be beneficial to pursue some experiments. What happens if we try such an approach? Perhaps the result is that the infant has difficulty cooperating and succeeding because he is not ready for this structured approach. Direct evidence of this may lead a parent to revise expectations, and be willing to explore alternative approaches. I find parents typically make choices in the best interest of the child. After observing what helps the child succeed, the parent may be willing to pursue other avenues to accomplish the desired goal.

The interventionist needs to realize that *it is important to watch, listen, and understand before advising, explaining, or instructing*. This is difficult if the sessions become too child-focused too soon. Time needs to be invested in listening to the parents, providing support, and in watching and supporting their interactions with the infant. I fondly recall a dad I worked with long ago whose toddler daughter contracted meningitis and was profoundly deaf. He was one of the best signers in our family sign class, but he had been unable to participate in many parent-infant sessions. One strategy I have used to become a partner with families is to work collaboratively to identify sign goals for themselves by jointly watching a videotape of their signed interaction with their child. Until I had a chance to watch Andy play with his daughter, I had no clue about how frustrated he was. He was able to sustain her visual attention for very brief periods. He spent a lot of time with attention getting strategies (like tapping her) that she ignored. Yet, there was one section on the tape where they took about ten successful conversational turns. He was following her lead effectively during this interaction in contrast to other parts where he was trying to introduce teaching episodes. We discussed his frustrations openly and then watched the successful section of the tape together. Through guided questioning, he discovered that what made the difference was his ability to follow his daughter's interests. I still remember his affect as he left my office that day. He had an "I can do this" attitude. That is really my point—we need to look for ways in intervention to support parents in discovering "I can do this!"

Basically, we are working to establish an even playing field—you have your expertise, I have mine. Together we can make an effective team for the benefit of the child and family. If we look at the history of parent/infant intervention, there has been a focus on professional modeling of effective techniques for families and requesting that they practice. There are times when this can be a successful tool, and parents indicate that they benefit from seeing models. It should be used cautiously, however, to avoid intervention that becomes a spectator sport.

Premise Three: Relationship-focused intervention in infancy supports caregiver-child reciprocity, social attachment, and recognition of and responsiveness to the child's communicative signals. This premise has to do with the developmental focus of intervention for the youngest of infants. It is interesting to reflect on some of the shifts that are occurring in early intervention practices as a result of Universal Newborn Hearing Screening efforts. In the past, many families came to early interventionists after lengthy delays in diagnosis. Such delays often left families feeling angry, guilty, and pressured to catch up as quickly as possible. Pressure to catch up sometimes resulted in parents attempting to be the child's teacher, which perhaps detracted from ability to gain joy from the relationship. Furthermore, interventionists were accustomed to working with somewhat older toddlers rather than newborns. Now we see a welcome shift toward earlier identifications through screening efforts. We are in a situation where parents can experience proactive management that seeks to prevent developmental consequences of hearing loss.

Some families of early-identified children respond with great relief that a concern in hearing was caught so early, putting them in a position to prevent communication delays. Now we encounter families who, as yet, may have little direct evidence that the baby cannot hear. In contrast to days of old where parents saw delays in speech and language and fought the system to address them, children identified through screening, especially those with milder losses, may show no visible signs of hearing loss. This may make it challenging for some families to understand hearing loss and its consequences for their baby, especially when they have evidence to the contrary. These represent new counseling challenges for professionals serving these families.

Some families find it hard to wait for visible signs of their efforts. Perhaps a family is eager for the child's first words, confirming that their pursuit of certain methods is in fact working. Parents of typically developing children also anxiously await first words, but with confidence that this development will unfold naturally. Parents of a child with hearing loss may be anxious for the child to produce words, so that they have evidence that what they are doing is addressing their child's needs. In addition to providing affective support, it is critical that early interventionists become well versed in infant development across various domains. In particular, families benefit when the provider helps them focus on developmentally appropriate stages in communication at the presymbolic level.

There are many useful resources from other disciplines that can be adapted for fostering interactions with deaf and hard-of-hearing babies. There are two practical resources that are useful in working with parents of very young infants. One set of resources has been developed by Dr. Stanley Greenspan. His text, *First Feelings*, introduces parents of babies to the early emotional development of infants. It offers guidance for promoting attachment and reciprocity through daily caregiving routines. For the infant aged up to eight months, direction focuses on shared attention and engagement, what Greenspan calls the first of six emotional milestones in childhood. At the shared attention and engagement stage, developmental expectations for the parent-infant dyad are listed in table II.

A second resource is a communication assessment tool that can be used to examine presymbolic and early symbolic attainments of infants 9 to 24 months of age. The Communication and Symbolic Behavior Scales (CSBS; Wetherby and Prizant 1993) is a semi-structured observational procedure that uses enjoyable strategies to "tempt" communication from an infant during semi-structured play interactions with parent and interventionist. It results in a profile of communicative functions typically observed in young infants, along with an accounting of the various preverbal and verbal communicative means a child has at his or her disposal. We have found this to be helpful in guiding parents in the identification of many behaviors such as communication, and in helping them wait for first words. This scale focuses the clinician's attention on the reciprocity of the parent-child relationship and on the development of social-affective signaling between partners. The tool also includes measures of language comprehension and play. The resulting profile of skills allows parents and interventionists to identify relative strengths and needs within the child's communicative profile, which assists with program planning and feeling hopeful and successful about what is being accomplished. In a way, it is helping families look at the glass half full, instead of focusing on "down the road" skills.

Table II. Skills of the parent-child dyad defined by Greenspan in the birth to eight month period of shared attention and engagement (Greenspan and Greenspan 1985).

Child Accomplishments	Caregiver Accomplishments
▪ The child is able to attend to multisensory affective experiences, organize a calm, regulated state and experience pleasure.	▪ Caregivers are attuned to the child's signals.
▪ The child is able to engage caregivers, express affective preferences, and show pleasure in interaction with caregivers.	▪ Caregivers make effective accommodations for the child's needs and abilities.
▪ The child has full access to conversations with caregivers.	▪ Caregivers nurture engagement and mutually satisfying shared experiences.
	▪ Caregivers see competence in the child and themselves during interactions.

Premise Four: In an empowerment model, we identify strengths that are present in each situation. It can be challenging to see strengths in certain situations, especially in family systems that are quite different from our own families. We must work to understand our own biases and perceptions as these can mask our ability to see unique strengths. Strengths may exist in forms we are not accustomed to exploring. There may be strengths in a family's value system that allows them to cope and adjust in unique ways. They may show competencies or abilities that can be recruited in the intervention process (e.g., a dad that was skilled at carpentry built a standing table for his son; he took pride in this contribution). We may also identify strengths in interactional and parenting skills. It is important for teams to focus on broad areas of potential strength.

Premise Five: Early intervention programs should strive to involve fathers. When there are developmental concerns for a child, roles can become tightly defined in families, with the mother becoming the primary caregiver and the father maintaining his role as provider (Davis and May 1991). It appears that many systems come to expect that fathers will be less involved. This may be a notion that interferes with meeting fathers' needs. According to one author who is a father of two health-impaired girls (Davis and May 1991), the medical and educational system reinforced this role definition in his case. He described how professionals expected him to be strong, to need less emotional support than his wife, and to be able to hold things together. He experienced a pronounced lack of support for his own emotional needs. He added that he envied the emotional support offered to women by female therapists, nurses, and teachers. He discovered that friends in the workplace did not want to listen to his concerns. His best support was the friendship of another father of a child with disabilities (Davis and May 1991). His comments reinforce the need to define family broadly enough when identifying sources of support. Table III includes helpful direction from these authors for involving fathers in early intervention.

I was curious about the ways that these traditional role definitions might be influencing paternal participation in our own program, and began to interview fathers about their perceptions. Several fathers stressed that it was natural and somewhat necessary in their families for the mother to take the lead in meeting the communicative needs of the child. However, I got a sense from each of them that the mothers and fathers saw themselves as a team working to meet the needs of the child. They capitalized on each others' strengths to meet the needs of the child and family as a whole. These fathers stressed that parent-to-parent contact was helpful to them, especially in informal settings. Not all wanted this in the form of father's groups. One father noted,

Table III. Strategies for Involving Men.

1.	Define a child's family as those persons who physically and emotionally touch the child through the care they offer. The expectation from professionals then can be that all family members are important to the child and all share the common goal of improving the life of the child and family. Decision-making relative to the child's care can then become a process where information can be shared, alternatives developed and decisions made in collaboration with families, not just the professional and the child's mother.
2.	Want and seek male involvement. This is the first and most effective step that can be made to develop programs that result in more meaningful participation by men.
3.	Review all aspects of existing programs from policy to implementation and determine if barriers are present which discourage or even punish male involvement.
4.	Adapt expectations that fathers will be participants in decisions involved in daily treatment and care of their children, and the child's and families' lives will be enriched by the participation.
5.	Don't assume men don't want to be involved: they do, but sometimes they don't know how. Show them a variety of ways to be involved and then support their involvement.
6.	Help hospital and clinical staff to understand the crucial importance of and facilitate male parent-to-parent contact.
7.	Assist service providers in directing medical/educational activities towards fathers as well as mothers. Sensitize them to assumptions they may have about rigid role definitions for men as decision makers and providers.
8.	Create fathers' support programs. Effective models exist: they need increased implementation.
9.	Offer training to professionals and staff by fathers.
10.	Involve men in all aspects of program development from policy to implementation.
11.	Incorporate what has been learned from fathers into curriculum and in service programs for staff and professionals.

Reprinted with permission from: Davis, P. and May, J. Involving fathers in early intervention and family support programs: Issues and strategies. *CHC* 20:2:87–92.

"Oh man, if you get a bunch of guys together we'd all be checking our watches and our Palm Pilots." I was reminded again to listen to families and to fathers as a way to understand their needs from us.

In closing, I reflect again on this exciting but complex era ahead. As interventionists, we are challenged to work with very young infants who come from families with diverse cultural backgrounds. We work to develop increased multi-cultural understanding and sensitivity. We search for resources in multiple languages to meet needs. We also serve many children with multiple disabilities, which taxes our developmental knowledge and requires that we devote time to cultivating transdisciplinary skills and perspectives. I have often observed that parent/infant situations require the most skilled providers. So, we, just like the families we work with, need staying power. Power to sustain our curiosity, innovation, and support for families over the long haul. This observation leads me to a final timeless lesson from David Luterman. I remember as a young clinician wondering why David Luterman went running with members of his parent group. I was too naïve to understand that he was modeling for parents the need for balance in one's life. Dennis McLoughlin, a teacher who has devoted his career to inspiring creativity in teaching, developed an acronym—ARFF—that relates to achieving a balance in our daily lives Achievement, Respect, Fun, and Freedom (McLoughlin 1999). He claims ARFF is something we need each day, just like a car needs four tires full of air. If one of the tires is low, the car is hard to drive. By Achievement, he means we can feel some success as a result of our efforts. We feel Respected when we have evidence that others listen to us and treat us with love and caring. Fun is obvious, but are we and families we work with taking time for it on a regular basis? Freedom refers to having the time to get our needs met—some flexibility in our schedules instead of a pileup of demands. For parents, it may be the freedom to make their own choices and the freedom to respond humanly to difficult experiences. As we embark on this promising era, we will do well to remember the timeless lessons from David Luterman that teach us to respond sensitively and humanely as we work to make a difference for families.

REFERENCES

American Academy of Pediatrics 1999. Newborn and infant hearing loss: Detection and intervention task force on newborn and infant hearing. *Pediatrics* 103:527–30.

Bailey, D. 1995. Personal communication.

Bailey, D. 1987. Collaborative goal-setting with families: Resolving differences in values and priorities for service. *Topics in Early Childhood Special Education* 7(2):59–71.

Bess F. H., and Paradise, J. L. 1994. Universal screening for infant hearing impairment: Not simple, not risk-free, not necessarily beneficial, and not presently justified. *Pediatrics* 93:330–34.

Blair, J., Peterson, M., and Viehweg, S. 1985. The effects of mild sensorineural hearing loss on academic performance of young school-age children. *Volta Review* 87:87–93.

Blank, M., Rose, S., and Berlin, L. 1978. *Preschool Language Assessment Instrument*. New York: Grune and Stratton.

Calderon, R. 2000. Parental involvement in deaf children's education programs as a predictor of child's language, early reading, and social-emotional development. *Journal of Deaf Studies and Deaf Education* 5 (2):140–55.

Calderon, R., Bargones, J., and Sidman, S. 1998. Characteristics of hearing families and their young deaf and hard of hearing children. *American Annals of the Deaf* 143(4):347–62.

Calderon, R., and Greenberg, M. 1997. The effectiveness of early intervention for deaf children and children with hearing loss. In *The Effectiveness of Early Intervention*, ed. M. J. Guralnick. Baltimore: Paul H. Brookes.

Calderon, R., and Low, S. 1998. Early social-emotional, language and academic development in children with hearing loss: Families with and without fathers. *AAD* 143:225–34.

Carney, A. E. 1996. Early intervention and management of the infant with hearing loss: What's science got to do with it? *Seminars in Hearing* 17:185–95.

Condon, M. C. 1997. A collaborative problems solving approach to early intervention. Workshop presented in Toronto, Canada.

Cross, T. G., Nienhuys, T. G., and Kirkman, M. 1985. Parent-child interaction with receptively disabled children: Some determinants of maternal speech style. In *Children's Language*, ed. K. E. Nelson. Hillsdale, NJ: Lawrence Erlbaum Associates.

Davis, F. B. 1942. Two new measures of reading ability. *Journal of Educational Psychology* 33:365–72.

Davis, J. M., Elfenbein, J. L., Schum, R., and Bentler, R. 1986. Effects of mild and moderate hearing impairments on language, educational, and psychosocial behavior of children. *Journal of Speech and Hearing Disorders* 51:53–62.

Davis, P. M., and May, J. E. 1991. Involving fathers in early intervention and family support programs: Issues and strategies. *Children's Health Care* 20(2):87–92.

Dromi, E., and Ingber, S. 1999. Israeli mothers' expectations from early intervention with their preschool deaf children. *Journal of Deaf Studies and Deaf Education* 4(1):50–68.

Dunn, L., and Dunn, L.1981. *Peabody Picture Vocabulary Test -Revised Manual.* Circle Pines, MN: American Guidance Service.

Family Enablement Project 1991. Workshop on Family Centered Practices.

Gallaway, C., and Woll, B. 1994. Interaction and childhood deafness. In *Input and Interaction in Language Acquisition*, eds. C. Gallaway and B. J. Richards. New York: Cambridge University Press.

Greenspan, S., and Greenspan, N. 1985. *First Feelings.* New York: Viking Press.

Guralnick, M. J. 1997. Second generation research in the field of early intervention. In *The Effectiveness of Early Intervention*, ed. M. Guralnick. Baltimore: Paul H. Brookes.

Hall, G., and Loucks, S. 1978. Teacher concerns as a basis for facilitating and personalizing staff development. *Teacher College Record* 80(1).

Joint Committee on Infant Hearing 1994. Joint Committee on Infant Hearing Position Statement. American Speech-Language-Hearing Association 36:38–41.

Koester, L. S., and Papousek, H. 2000. Intuitive parenting, communication, and interaction with deaf infants. In *The Deaf Child in the Family and School*, eds. P. Spencer, C. Erting, and M. Marschark. Mahwah, NJ: Lawrence Erlbaum and Associates.

Koester, L. S., Karwoski, A. M., and Traci, M. A. 1998. How do deaf and hearing mothers regain eye contact when their infants look away? *AAD* 143:5–13.

Lederberg, A., and Prezbindowski, A. 2000. Impact of child deafness on mother-toddler interaction: Strengths and weaknesses. In *The Deaf Child in the Family and School*, eds. P. Spencer, C. Erting, and M. Marschark. Mahwah, NJ: Lawrence Erlbaum and Associates.

Levitt, H., and McGarr, N. 1988. Speech and language development in hearing-impaired children. In *Hearing Impairment in Children*, ed. F. H. Bess. Timonium, MD: York Press.

Mahoney, G., Boyce, G., Fewell, R., Spiker, D. and Wheeden, C. A. 1998. The relationship of parent-child interaction to the effectiveness of early intervention services for at-risk children and children with disabilities. *Topics in Early Childhood Special Education* 18 (1):5–17.

McBride, S. L. and Peterson, C. 1997. Home-based intervention with families of children with disabilities: Who is doing what? *Topics in Early Childhood Special Education* 17(2): 209–33.

McLoughlin, D. 1999. High Trust Psychology. http://www.hightrust.net.

Mertens, D., Sass-Lehrer, M., and Scott-Olson, K. 2000. Sensitivity in the family-professional relationship: Parental experiences in families with young deaf and hard of hearing children. In *The Deaf Child in the Family and School*, eds. P. Spencer, C. Erting, and M. Marschark. Mahwah, NJ: Lawrence Erlbaum and Associates.

Moeller, M. P. 2000. Early intervention and language outcomes in children who are deaf and hard of hearing. *Pediatrics* 106, 3(e43): 1–9.

Moeller, M. P., and Condon, M. 1994. A collaborative, problem-solving approach to early intervention. In *Infants and Toddlers with Hearing Loss: Identification, Assessment and Family-Centered Intervention*, eds. J. Roush and N. D. Matkin. Timonium, MD: York Press.

Moeller, M. P., and Condon, M. 1998. Family Matters: Making sense of complex choices. In *Children with Hearing Impairment: Contemporary Trends*, ed. F. Bess. Nashville, TN: Vanderbilt Bill Wilkerson Center Press.

Moeller, M. P., Donaghy, K. F., Beauchaine, K. L., Lewis, D. E., and Stelmachowicz, P. G. 1996. Longitudinal study of FM system use in non-academic settings: Effects on language development. *Ear and Hearing* 17:28–41.

Moeller, M. P., Osberger, M. J., McConkey, A. J., and Eccarius, M. A. 1981. Some language skills of the students in a residential school for the deaf. *Journal of the Academy of Rehabilitative Audiology* 14:84–111.

Mohay, H. 2000. Language in sight: Mothers' strategies for making language visually accessible to deaf children. In *The Deaf Child in the Family and School*, eds. P. Spencer, C. Erting, and M. Marschark. Mahwah, NJ: Lawrence Erlbaum and Associates.

NIH Consensus Statement 1993. Identification of Hearing Impairment in Infants and Young Children 11:1–24. Bethesda, MD: NIH.

Reynell, J. K. 1977. *Reynell Developmental Language Scales.* Windsor, England: NFER Publishing Company.

Schilling, R. F., Kirkham, M. S., Snow, W. H., and Schnike, S. 1986. Single mothers with handicapped children: Different from their married counterparts? *Family Relations* 35:69–77.

Schuyler, V., and Rushmer, N. 1987. *Parent-infant Habilitation: A Comprehensive Approach to Working with Hearing-impaired Infants and Toddlers and Their Families.* Portland: IHR Publications.

Spencer, P., and Lederberg, A. R. 1998. Different modes, different models: Communication and language of young deaf children and their mothers. In *Communication and Language Acquisition: Discoveries from Atypical Development*, eds. L. B. Adamson and M.A. Romski. Baltimore: Paul H. Brookes.

Watkins, S., Pittman, P., and Walden, B. 1998. The deaf mentor experimental project for young deaf children who are deaf and their families. *AAD* 143(1):29–34.

Wetherby, A., and Prizant, B. 1993. Communication and Symbolic Behavior Scales. *Applied Symbolix*, 800 N. Wells, Suite 200, Chicago, IL, 60610.

Yoshinaga-Itano, C., Sedey, A. L., Coulter, B. A., and Mehl, A. L. 1998. Language of early-and later-identified children with hearing loss. *Pediatrics* 102(5):1168–71.

Zimmerman, I., Steiner, V., and Pond, R.1992. *Preschool Language Scale - 3.* San Antonio, TX: The Psychological Corp.

Chapter ■ 9

Professional Training in Audiology: *Past, Present, and Future*

Fred H. Bess

It is a privilege for me to participate in a volume that honors one of the giants of our profession, David Luterman. Few in the profession, past or present, have contributed more to children with hearing impairment and their families.

This chapter reflects on the professional training of audiologists, especially those audiologists working with children. To this end, the chapter offers an overview on professional training from a historical perspective, beginning with our past educational efforts, reviewing the present day status of professional training, and then proffering some comments on training needs for the future.

PROFESSIONAL TRAINING IN THE PAST

The discipline of audiology evolved during Word War II—a time when Army and Naval hospitals were serving more than 16,000 war-deafened military personnel (Bess and Humes 1995). Following the war, professional training programs in audiology evolved at a rapid pace beginning at several major universities across the country—Iowa, Northwestern, and Stanford to name only a few.

This was the early infant stage of audiology. Most training programs were housed in departments of speech and theater, or occasionally, special education. Many audiology training programs had only one faculty member. During this early period, the vast majority of audiologists were employed in hospital settings or universities, and the focus of the profession tended to be medical. That is, the emphasis was on assessment, diagnosis, and using special auditory tests to identify lesions along the auditory pathways. Tests such as difference limens, Bekesy patterns, and tone decay provided the "buzz" words of the day.

Audiology quickly expanded its scope of practice to amplification, screening, habilitation, and rehabilitation. The average age of identification for hearing impairment in children was four to five years. Hearing aids were large, unattractive, provided a limited bandwidth, and generated high levels of harmonic distortion (Ross 1996; Killion 1997). Assessment procedures relied on sound field and play audiometry. The procedures for selecting a hearing aid were limited and often it took as long as six months to one year to finalize the hearing aid fitting. During the lengthy fitting process, Y-cords were often used to ensure that each ear received some amount of auditory stimulation (Bess 2000).

Not surprisingly, the course work in audiology was limited in those early years. A general outline of a course of study for a trainee in 1961 is shown in table I. The course of study spanned three semesters and 15 hours were in clinical audiology. Moreover, the student received fewer than 200 hours of clinical practice. Importantly, only one

Table I. Course of Study for an Audiology Graduate Student Obtaining the Master's Degree in 1961

Fall	Hours	Spring	Hours	Summer	Hours
Anatomy and Function of the Speech and Hearing Mechanism	3	Voice Science	3	Statistics	4
Speech and Language Development of the Acoustically Handicapped	3	Organic Speech Disorders	4	Speechreading	3
Psychology of Deafness	3	Stuttering	3	Diagnosis and Appraisal	3
Introduction to Audiology	3	Advanced Audiology	3		
	12		13		10

Total Practicum Hours 195

course focused on the pediatric population. Students were seldom exposed to children with hearing loss and their families. There were no courses on counseling, hearing aids, pediatric assessment, or habilitation/rehabilitation. In fact, most audiologists were uncomfortable working with children, and especially with their families. Such discomfort was directly linked to the limited educational experiences students received with young children and their families.

There were very few audiology textbooks available to the profession. Perhaps the most popular text was *Audiology* (Newby 1958), an introduction to the practice of audiology. Other textbooks used during this period included *Auditory Disorders in Children* (Mykelbust 1954), *Hearing and Deafness* (Davis and Silverman 1960), and *The Psychology of Deafness* (Mykelbust 1960).

In 1952, the American Speech-Language-Hearing Association (ASHA) developed a certification program designed to set minimum academic and clinical standards for entering the profession of audiology. There were two levels of certification, basic and advanced. In basic certification, the audiologist was required to take a total of 30 semester hours—at least 12 hours in audiology and three hours in speech-language pathology. An advanced certification was attainable for those individuals who obtained a total of 60 semester hours of course work, at least 21 hours in audiology, and six to nine hours in speech-language pathology. Four hundred hours of practicum were required followed by four years of sponsored professional experience. Advanced certification also required passing a written and oral examination.

In 1965, the profession moved to a single level of certification. Applicants were required to show evidence of a master's degree or equivalent, 60 semester hours of course work, 275 hours of practicum, completion of nine months of supervised practicum, a letter from the director of a graduate program, and a passing score on a national examination.

PROFESSIONAL TRAINING IN THE PRESENT

Predictably, present day audiology requirements are much more stringent. Today, an audiology student must exhibit 75 semester hours of course work, 30 hours of which will focus on various aspects of clinical audiology, six hours in speech-language pathology, and no fewer than 375 clock hours in clinical practice. A student will typically complete a 36-week clinical fellowship under direct supervision and achieve a passing score on a national examination. Such a course of study will usually require five semesters of academic course work and related practicum.

DEVELOPMENTS AND CHALLENGES THAT HAVE AN IMPACT ON TRAINING PROGRAMS

In recent years, several developments have evolved to influence and challenge our current day training programs. First, we have come to recognize that the demographics of children with hearing impairment have changed. Today, audiologists are being asked to serve a distinctively different group of children with hearing loss than those we served in the 1960s and 1970s. That is, a shift has taken place in the prevalence of causation and the prevalence of degree of hearing loss. Because of improved health care we no longer see some of the major factors that result in severe to profound sensorineural hearing loss—causes such as maternal ruebella, hemolytic disease, and ototoxicity. Instead, we are witnessing a host of etiologies that produce milder forms of hearing loss. Conditions such as prenatal disease, new forms of hereditary deafness, middle ear disease, and noise from leisure activities are all known to produce milder forms of hearing impairment. We do not know the prevalence of these milder forms of hearing loss, however, we do know that the milder the loss, the higher the prevalence. Such demographic changes have important implications for training educators and audiologists to meet the documented needs of children with mild hearing impairments.

Legislative initiatives have also had a strong influence on training institutions. Since the passage of Public Law 99-457, The Education of the Handicapped Act Amendments of 1986, unprecedented expansion of services have been brought to infants, toddlers, and preschool children with disabilities and their families. All 50 states and outlying territories now provide services for infants and toddlers with disabilities through Part C of the 1997 Re-authorization of IDEA. Children with disabilities aged three to five are served under Part B of IDEA. As a result of the expanded Child Find efforts, it is predicted that more than 700,000 young children with disabilities and their families will need services in fiscal year 98/99 (Bureau of Census 1997). The growth rate for the number of young children with disabilities aged birth to five years from 1993/94 to 1994/95 was almost twice the growth rate for services for children six to eighteen years (18th Annual Report to Congress 1997). Hence, these initiatives have created an urgent need to train high quality early childhood specialists and early interventionists. Indeed, personnel in all areas of special education are needed who have specialized skills in working with families, as well as with children, and in collaborating with personnel from other disciplines to plan and conduct child interventions.

One of the goals for Healthy People 2000 and 2010 is to reduce the average age of identification for hearing loss by 12 months or fewer. Consequently, we have witnessed an increased emphasis on early identification of hearing loss in children. Presently, 32 states mandate newborn hearing screening in the United States; more than 150 universal newborn hearing screening programs are currently in operation (ASHA, Personal Communication). Such a focus on early identification has resulted in a significant increase in the number of infants and toddlers referred to audiologists for early audiologic management and intervention services. Unfortunately, most audiologists do not have the appropriate training or the experiences to provide young infants and toddlers with proper assessment and management of hearing loss.

In the decades of the 80s and 90s, the profession of audiology underwent an explosion of evolving technology that expanded our scope of practice to such areas as cochlear implants, assistive devices, diagnostic, and management procedures. Because much of this technology was new and evolving, it was not well represented in the curriculum of training institutions designed to educate students in audiology.

Finally, it is important to emphasize that health care has changed dramatically in the last 20 years. We have witnessed dramatic changes in the way in which audiology is practiced and hearing health care is delivered. Contributing to these changes have been technological developments, increasing regulation of the entire health care industry, social change, changes in the organization of general health care delivery, changing priorities, and changes in the mechanism for financing health care. All of these factors have exerted significant influence on the utilization of hearing health care services. Hence, educational programs must inform students about the "real world" changes in health care and how such changes have influenced the practice of audiology. Moreover, we must recognize that a new paradigm for practicing audiology has emerged through health care reform, one that is more evidence based (Bess 2000).

Indeed, many of these changes and challenges have resulted in national shortages for professionals who work in special education. According to a recent national survey (Department of Education 1999), there were 246 vacancies for teachers of the hearing impaired, 2,501 vacancies in speech-language pathology, and 50 vacancies in educational audiology. If one considers those children between three and six years of age, the shortage data increases significantly.

NEEDS IN PROFESSIONAL TRAINING

One way to assess the effectiveness of training programs is to examine the practice behaviors and patterns of today's clinical audiologists. In this regard, one finds that training gaps can be identified in the areas of evaluation, amplification, special populations, counseling, and early intervention.

Evaluation

Survey studies have demonstrated that many audiologists are inadequately prepared for conducting comprehensive diagnostic evaluations, especially with children. Jacobson and colleagues (1998;1990) reported that only half the training programs surveyed believed graduates were competent in the area of auditory evoked potentials. Moreover, only 7% of the practicing audiologists considered themselves sufficiently competent to include auditory-evoked potentials in their assessment battery.

Amplification

Similar findings have been reported in the area of amplification. For example, Hedley-Williams and colleagues (1996) surveyed a large number of audiologists serving young children. This survey revealed that there was no systematic procedure used with children for fitting hearing aids. In general, recommended prescriptive procedures for hearing aid selection are not being used, probe tube measurements are typically not included as part of the verification strategy (aided sound field is the method of choice), and programmable hearing aids and assistive devices are seldom selected for children. Tharpe (2000) reported similar findings. Given the above findings, it is not surprising to note that training programs afford graduate students with limited educational experiences in fitting children with hearing aids. Most programs offer only one course in pediatrics (Bess 2000), while 18% of the programs offer nothing whatsoever. Hence, students rarely, if ever, receive exposure to fitting young infants and toddlers with hearing aids. In addition, they receive almost no exposure to the wide array of assistive listening devices available for young children with hearing impairment.

We also find a void in the training preparation of students in the area of cochlear implants. Approximately 8,000 children have received implants in the United States, and this number is projected to increase by 20% per year (Advanced Bionics, Personal Communication). Moreover, when surveying the top 20 programs in audiology and speech-language pathology, only one program in speech and two in audiology offer a course on implants. Similar findings were obtained when surveying deaf education programs (Teris Schery, personal communication). None of the programs offer information about cochlear implants from a multidisciplinary/transdisciplinary perspective—an interesting finding when one considers that the management of children with hearing loss who have implants centers around a multidisciplinary approach.

Finally, it is important to note that audiologists receive limited exposure to hearing impaired children with additional handicaps. It is estimated that some 30% to 40% of children with hearing impairment have at least one other handicapping condition. Nevertheless, only 32% of pediatric audiologists received at least one lecture on children with additional handicaps, and 19% received instruction on hearing aid fitting of children with such handicaps (Tharpe 2000). Perhaps the most important finding from the survey by Tharpe (2000) is that, irrespective of the type of additional handicapping condition (visual impairment, mental retardation, physical impairment, autism), the hearing aid fitting procedure and selection of microphone type are essentially the same. That is, we do not alter our selection procedures based on type of handicapping condition or conditions the child might have.

Special Populations

We also note that preparation programs fail to familiarize students in the identification, assessment, and management of children with central auditory processing disorders (CAPD). In general, it is reported that there exist more than 60 different tools used in CAPD assessment (Nelson and Bess 1998). Some of the difficulties with CAPD include: (1) no agreement on the pass/fail criterion; (2) no agreement on method of treatment; (3) inadequate training in the area of CAPD; and, (4) inadequate training to conduct rehabilitation for children diagnosed with CAPD.

Similar findings are found among children with autism. Only 33% of the speech-language pathologists surveyed in the southeast region exhibited any course work on autism in undergraduate or graduate training. Seventy-five percent of the speech pathologists felt that their training was inadequate. None of the audiologists surveyed throughout the southeast region had ever had a course in autism.

Counseling

With regard to counseling, we also find problems in preparation of audiologists, especially as it pertains to infants and toddlers and their families. According to a survey by Culpepper and colleagues (1994), only 12% of the United States training programs in communication disorders offer course work and practicum in counseling. Many audiologists in the United States feel ill-prepared to counsel parents of young children with hearing impairment. In studies by Crandell and colleagues (1996) and Crandell (1997), half of the audiology programs surveyed devoted less than 10% of a lecture time for counseling in hearing aid classes. Moreover, only about half of the programs offer a course in counseling. The majority of the programs expect students to obtain their counseling skills from clinical activities. In the words of Luterman and Kurtzer-White (1999), "with the number of hearing/ screening programs rapidly expanding, highly trained professionals with parent counseling skills are at a premium, as are specialists skilled in working with infants with hearing loss and their families."

Early Intervention

Finally, there is an important need to provide greater focus on early audiologic management and intervention within our training programs. Recall that legislation mandates education to begin attending to children at the infant and toddler age. One impact of this law is the need to train pediatric audiologists on the current issues, theories, and rehabilitation processes of hearing, speech, or language impaired infants and toddlers. In general, university programs emphasize educational training for populations above the toddler age; rarely do audiologists receive preparation on effective techniques for working with very young children. Oyler and Matkin (1987) surveyed 200 certified audiologists and found that over 30% believed they had insufficient training to work with young children. A large number of the respondents received fewer than five hours of supervised practicum with neonates and infants. Deaf education programs also fail to prepare teachers adequately to work with younger age groups. Fewer than half of deaf education programs offer training in early intervention (Roush et al. 1994).

PROFESSIONAL TRAINING IN THE FUTURE

What then is the future of professional training for our profession? Although we have clearly made important progress in our attempts to prepare professionals to work effectively with children and their families, we must continue to improve the professional training of audiologists. How we best achieve this goal, however, is the subject of much discussion and disagreement. Whatever these discussions and disagreements, it is clear to most of us that a change is needed and that the professional doctorate or the Au.D. should become the entry level requirement for the practitioner. There is no need here to offer the rationale or present the arguments for the professional doctorate. Such arguments have been made many times and have appeared in numerous professional and trade journals. Suffice it to say that most of the arguments, but certainly not all of them, are credible and persuasive to those of us in the profession. Accordingly, all professional organizations associated with audiology have endorsed the professional doctorate as the entry level credential for the practice of audiology. A degree which allows for additional years of study should facilitate the preparation of highly qualified personnel to serve very young children with hearing disabilities and their families.

Of great concern is the diminishing number of Ph.D.s in our profession, especially those in academia. Ph.D. graduates in audiology for 1997/98 ($N = 14$) and 1998/99 ($N = 8$) were the lowest number since 1982. In addition, there are more academic positions in communication disorders than there are graduates to fill them. It is important to note that of those Ph.D.s graduating in communication disorders, at least one half will pursue careers in the private sector. Finally, the average age of Ph.D.s in the profession is 59, hence in the next ten to twelve years about one half of our Ph.D. pool in academia will retire. We thus have a situation in which there is a shrinking number of Ph.D.s pursuing careers in communication disorders—for those who do elect a career in our profession, smaller numbers are entering academia. Who will train the next generation of audiologists? Who will conduct the important research to improve our identification, assessment, and management procedures? Who will generate the new knowledge in our profession for maintaining professional status and integrity?

Also, there is a need to improve research training in our educational programs. In the past decade there has been a steady decrease in the scientific basis for audiology. Research represents the primary mechanism for improving our services to individuals with hearing handicaps. It is through research that we develop new knowledge leading to improved methods of evaluation, treatment, rehabilitation, and prevention. Without a genuine commitment to a strong scientific basis upon which to structure new developments in clinical service delivery, our professional services will weaken to a point where other professions will gradually assume our role. Hence, we must strengthen the research training of all our professionals. Audiologists on the Ph.D. level must have a firm understanding of the scientific method. They must be trained to be critical thinkers, continually questioning and challenging the basis of time-honored practices, procedures, and philosophies. They must be inspired to be creative thinkers constantly seeking improved methods through innovative and imaginative investigation. We must be ever mindful that if our students of today are to carry the profession forward for the future, they must be given a complete in-depth preparation of what is now, and trained, motivated, even inspired to think toward what will be tomorrow. Hence, the most important contribution one can make to the future development of audiology is to prepare the young mind, inspired and excited by the challenges and rewards of the profession. The rewards of the future depend on how well we meet the challenges of the present. Today is what we have learned, tomorrow is what we can teach.

REFERENCES

Bess, F. H. 2000. Early amplification for children: Implementing change. In *A Sound Foundation through Early Amplification*, ed. R. Seewald. Proceedings of an International Conference.

Bess, F. H., and Humes, L. E. 1995. *Audiology: The Fundamentals*, 2nd ed., Baltimore, MD: Williams and Wilkins.

Crandell, C. C. 1997. An update on counseling instruction within audiology programs. *The Journal of the Academy of Rehabilitative Audiology* 30:77–86.

Crandell, C. C., McDermott, D. J., and Pugh, K. 1996. A survey in amplification and counseling skills in audiology. *The Hearing Review* 3:26–29.

Culpepper, N. B., Mendel, L. L., and McCarthy, P. A. 1994. Counseling experience and training offered by ESB-accredited programs: An update. *ASHA* 36:55–58.

Davis, H., and Silverman, S. R. 1960. *Hearing and Deafness.* New York: Holt, Rinehart, and Winston.

Hedley-Williams, A., Tharpe, A. M., and Bess, F. H. 1996. Fitting hearing aids in children: A survey of practice procedures. *In Amplification for Children With Auditory Deficits*, eds. F. H. Bess, J. S. Gravel, and A. M. Tharpe. Nashville, TN: Bill Wilkerson Center Press.

Killion, M. C. 1997. Hearing aids: Past, present and future: Moving toward normal conversations in noise. *British Journal of Audiology* 31:141–8.

Luterman, D. M., and Kurtzer-White, E. 1999. *The Young Deaf Child.* Timonium, MD: York Press.

Myklebust, H. R. 1960. *The Psychology of Deafness.* New York: Grune and Stratton.

Myklebust, H. R. 1954. *Auditory Disorders in Children.* New York: Grune and Stratton.

Nelson, D., and Bess, F. H. 1998. Clinical practices in CAPD: Results from an international survey. Poster session presented at the American Academy of Audiology annual convention, Los Angeles: CA. Supported by the American Academy of Audiology New Investigators Research Award.

Newby, H. A. 1958. *Audiology: Principles and Practice.* New York: Appleton-Centry-Crofts, Inc.

Oyler, R., and Matkin, N. 1987.

Ross, M. 1996. Amplification for children: The process begins. In *Amplification for Children with Auditory Deficits*, eds. F. H. Bess, J. S. Gravel, and A. M. Tharpe. Nashville, TN: Bill Wilkerson Center Press.

Roush, J., Harrison, M., Palsha, S., and Davidson, D. 1994. *American Annals of the Deaf* 137:425–30.

Tharpe, A. M. 2000. Service delivery for children with multiple impairments: How are we doing? In *A Sound Foundation Through Early Amplification*, ed. R. Seewald. Proceedings of an International Conference.

Chapter ▪ 10

Closing Remarks

David Luterman

When my very precocious daughter was five years old, she asked me, "What was the best thing that ever happened to you?" Of course the only answer I could give her was "the day you were born." She persisted, as was her wont, and after we went through the birth of her siblings, I answered that I hoped it had not happened yet. After the two days of this marvelous symposium, I think it may have happened! I want to thank everybody for organizing and making the symposium possible; it has been a very special time for me. It feels to me as though my whole life has been in preparation for this moment. My fear is that it is going to be all downhill from here.

For me, working at Emerson has been a remarkable experience—one that I never anticipated. After working for five years developing the clinic, it occurred to me in a blinding epiphany that I really hated doing audiology. I knew this was true when I began to hope that patients would not show up. Prior to that time I was desperately trying to find them. So, I began looking for ways to extricate myself from doing clinical audiology while remaining at Emerson, where I was very happy.

When I was a graduate student at Penn State, there was a summer program for families in which there was a child suspected of having a hearing loss. The families were invited to attend the camp for a week of diagnostic evaluations and speech and language therapy. The clinicians in the program were selected from the graduate students. I was involved with that program for two years as a graduate assistant and Cari, my wife, was the nursery school teacher. For the duration of the program, we literally lived with the parents of newly diagnosed deaf children. I can see now that that was the most significant learning event of my entire graduate training. It is my fondest hope that the current nursery is also a fertile field for students in training and has had a similar effect on them.

That program became the prototype for my transition out of clinical audiology. I set about trying to get funding for the establishment of a nursery. The chair of our department at that time put me in touch with one of Emerson's trustees. (He also happened to be a trustee of a fund that was in the process of dissolving itself. Of such thin threads are careers and programs made!) John Lindsley was a Canadian uranium miner who had made and lost a series of fortunes. In one boom year, he established the Thayer Lindsley Fund with which to do philanthropic work in honor of his son who was killed in the second world war, and fortunately Lindsley tied the money up or he probably would have lost it. I submitted a grant proposal for $15,000 to the fund, basically for money to convert a garage into a nursery. At that time, the garage was used by the wrestling team and we had to evict them. I told my graduate assistant at that time that if any well-built young man came looking for me, to tell him I had left.

We stretched the $15,000 as far as we could, adding a room and converting the overhead door to a wall. We had to stint on the insulation and consequently we froze in the winter and baked in the summer. The facility lasted for over thirty years; recently we have moved into a new building with all the amenities, which works well, but totally lacks charm.

Cari and I went shopping for equipment, and although we didn't have much money we decided to buy quality goods, most of which are still in use 30 odd years later after having stood up to years of abuse by generations of deaf two-year olds. We opened the doors in 1965 with my wife, Cari, as the nursery school teacher and two of the college staff as communication therapists. Looking back on that marvelous time, I must admit that I did not know what I was doing other than knowing that I must involve the parents in everything that was happening. Unknown to me we had a rubella epidemic the year before and there was an enormous demand for our services. We had parents banging on the door to get in and at one point we had three groups going simultaneously. The parents in our first group were marvelous. They helped me through the first years and taught me a great deal. Many of them remain good friends to this day. I look back on what I did not know then and wonder how I ever had the "chutzpah" to have started that program. I think you have to be young and ignorant as I was, and perhaps also a bit desperate.

The next year I submitted a proposal to the Office of Education to fund the nursery for three years as a demonstration program, which we were awarded. At that time, I thought that I would just do this for the next three years and then figure out what I really wanted to do. Thirty-five years later I am still here. I guess I must be a little slow. The nursery has been an incredibly satisfying life work; I have never been bored by it and I am always being taught something new. And while the essentials of adapting to a catastrophic change in one's life remain the same, the way they play out within a family and within a group are infinite. Almost every parent group challenges me in some way.

This symposium affords me a unique opportunity to look at what I have learned over the past 40 years and perhaps to look ahead a bit. If we do not know where we have been, then we really cannot know where we are headed—our past is a stable compass for us. Our view of things is always a function of the time we lived in and where we sit. We are all prisoners of our own experience.

I feel very fortunate to have witnessed and participated in the huge advance in education of the deaf that has taken place over the past four decades. When I started in 1960, the outlook for a newly diagnosed deaf child was rather bleak. He or she could look forward to a rather restricted life with few options—speech was likely to be unintelligible, literacy minimal, and education was most likely in a school for the deaf. Social and vocational options were also very limited. I think, 40 years later, we have at hand all the tools necessary to eliminate the negative educational consequences of deafness. The newly diagnosed deaf child of the new millennium has many more possibilities than his or her counterpart of 40 years ago. He or she will probably be diagnosed at birth or shortly thereafter, fit with sophisticated amplification, and if the aids are not helpful, then with a cochlear implant. More likely than not, deaf children of today will be educated within the mainstream with normally hearing children. Whether or not they are happier than their counterparts of 40 years ago is problematic, and whether or not we as a profession intelligently apply everything we now know about early childhood deafness remains equally problematic.

I have predicated my career on the simple notion that the most expedient way to help a young deaf child is to help the parents, and therefore we should direct our programmatic thrust at the parents rather than the child. I have found it personally frustrating as I talk with other professionals working with young deaf children. They all say parents are important and they all do parent education. It is rare however, to find a program where the parent actually is the centerpiece. Most professionals are distracted by the child, and parents are usually relegated to a peripheral role. This model generally fits the professionals training, and to be fair the parents, inclinations. Yet , I believe, if we can keep the parent as our primary responsibility, especially in the early stages of diagnosis and therapy, all sorts of good things happen for the child.

Here are some of the things I have learned over the years:

You have to program for the parents. It is easy to get distracted by children; trying to append a parent program onto an essentially child-centered program does not work. Despite all the energy and polemics devoted to it, methodology is not the important issue. I think any method can work if consistently and competently applied. If I have learned anything over the past forty years of watching children, it is that they are immensely diverse in their communication needs and abilities. A "one size fits all" method cannot possibly work. The methodology wars have obscured the important issues in education of the deaf that have limited progress, namely, poor pedagogy, failure to use technology well, and the under utilization of parents.

An active, high self-esteeming parent will get language to the child by the best possible means. In short, it is the parent who will solve the methodology problem. Our job as professionals is to provide information and support to the parent. The monumental work of Schlesinger (1992), who found that the best predictor of literacy for a child was maternal self-esteem, is in total accord with my own experience. Any clinical procedure we employ must be evaluated in terms of whether or not it enhances maternal self-esteem.

Listening and valuing are the most helpful clinical interventions we can use. They are the means to enhance parental self-esteem. What diminishes parents is rescuing and over helping; what I have called the Annie Sullivan effect.

The parent support group is the primary vehicle for healing the pain of deafness for the hearing parent. It provides for the recognition of the universality of the feelings engendered by the diagnosis of deafness and attenuates the loneliness the parents feel. The precept that feelings just are—that parents need not be responsible for how they feel, only how they behave—is the most helpful construct for parents in the early stages of diagnosis, along with acceptance. I could not conceive of an early intervention program without a support group.

Deafness is a family affair. In order to be successful in our early intervention efforts we must extend our scope of practice to include siblings and grandparents. The longer I work with families the more I see that the family is a complex system with all of the parts intricately interconnected.

There is a great deal of pain in deafness and also a great deal of growth. Deafness is a teacher, if we allow it to function that way. It can and does bring out good qualities in both children and parents that might otherwise lie latent. I am often asked how I could stay amidst so much pain. I stay focused on the growth. I never pity parents, but I can empathize with the pain and rejoice with them in the growth.

To look ahead a bit: I am very concerned about the effects that universal screening of newborns has on the diagnostic process and on therapeutic interventions. In theory, I am not opposed to screening; in practice I am appalled at the results. It looks to me as though an unintended consequence of universal screening of newborns has been to remove the audiologist from making the initial diagnosis. In data we have gathered on parents of deaf children who have had their children screened, not one was seen initially by an audiologist. Instead they were informed of the screening failure by either a pediatrician, nurse, or technician, none of whom could provide the parents with any information. Most parents did not get to see an audiologist until at least a month had passed in order to get confirmation of the loss. By that time, in the words of one parent, "I was a total basket case." Horror stories abound: Parents finding out by overhearing giggling nurses, by seeing a note on the child's bassinet that he or she had failed the test, or being told by a nurse as they were leaving the hospital, "By the way, your child failed his hearing test, but don't worry about it."

We have discarded the typical parent-initiated model of diagnosis for an institution-initiated model without an awareness of the implications of this change. In the past it was the parent who slowly became aware of the child's failure to respond to sound. Often the parent encountered opposition from family, friends, and sometimes professionals. The diagnostic process for the audiologist was mainly one of confirming what the parent already knew. Thus, the audiologist was often viewed as an ally and the diagnosis was met with relief because it explained much of the child's aberrant behavior. The new diagnostic paradigm, however, presents a very different set of challenges. In the new institution-initiated model, unsuspecting parents who have just gone through the grueling birth process are told by an uninformed professional or quasi-professional that their child may be deaf. There is never a good time to tell parents that their child is deaf, but I can think of no worse time than one or two days post partum. People often slay the messenger when they don't like the message, and there are going to be many audiologists slaughtered in the wake of parental wrath. It does not seem to me that our profession is prepared to handle such a profound change in the parent/audiologist relationship.

Of equal concern to me is the failure of management. It is relatively easy to set up screening programs—it seems that it is much harder to have good follow up, as evidenced by the recently published appalling data that only 15% of children get fitted with amplification before three months of age and only fifteen percent receive therapy before six months of age (Arehart et al.). It looks to me that we are telling parents that they have a deaf child at birth and then leaving them without any supportive services. This cannot be in the child's or parents' best interests. It seems to me that any advantage that early detection would give is rapidly lost if there is not adequate follow up. In fact, we may be harming the child by interfering with the bonding that needs to take place for the child's psychological development by not providing parents with the necessary emotional support for them to accept their child's deafness.

Most audiologists after confirming the diagnosis and fitting the child with hearing aids seem to refer the family to an early intervention program, and thereafter have a very marginal role in the child's habilitation. Our experience has been that early intervention programs are rarely comfortable with a deaf child, let alone an infant. (Ellen Kurtzer-White has been accumulating data to this effect.) And I think it behooves us as professionals, to take more responsibility for the habilitative aftermath of an infant screening program. If we are enthusiastic about screening, then we need to be equally enthusiastic about the management component.

I think we are, by virtue of early detection and the application of currently available technology, stumbling our way toward creating a new kind of deaf child—one who will function as a hard-of-hearing child in the educational mainstream. What concerns me is that many of these children do not do well socially. While their academic achievements are usually impressive, certainly by previous standards, it is bought at a huge cost. These are not happy children. I have found that their success has been achieved at the painful price of social isolation, low self-esteem, and severe identity problems. This is why the deaf community becomes an appealing alternative to many of these "successful" oral adults. We are going to see many more of these children over the coming years, unless we start putting in place the necessary supporting structures so that these children can truly succeed. We are going to produce another generation of angry, unhappy deaf adults. We are going to need new educational paradigms, and I am not at all optimistic that this is occurring. The profession of audiology has tended to have a short-term focus and be technology driven. This is not necessarily very helpful to the clients we are pledged to serve.

For me, personally, as I look back on four decades of work, I feel truly blessed to have been of service and to have met so many marvelous people. My life has turned out far better than I ever thought possible, and I have to hope along with the poet Browning "that the best is yet to be." In fact, I have been having so much fun I am trying to figure out how I can "retire" again next year.

June 2, 2000

References

Arehart, K., Yoshinaga-Itano, C., Thomson, V., Gabbard, S., Brown, A.1998. State of states: The status of universal newborn hearing screening, assessment and intervention systems in 16 states. *American Journal of Audiology* 77(2):101–14.

Schlesinger, H. 1992.The elusive x-factor: Parental contributions to literacy. In *A Free hand*, eds. M. Walworth, D. Moores, and T.O. Rourke. Silver Spring, MD ; T. J Publishers.

Index

(Page numbers in italics indicate material in tables or figures)